Digestive Diseases

Clinical Reviews

Formerly 'Survey of Digestive Diseases'
Founded in 1983 by T.S.N. Chen and R.K. Zetterman
Former Editor: S.R. Achem (1993–2000)

KARGER

Printed in Switzerland on acid-free paper by Reinhardt Druck, Basel

Appears quarterly: 1 volume per year (4 issues)

Digestive Diseases

General Information

Publication data: 'Digestive Diseases' is published 4 times a year. Volume 19 with 4 issues appears in 2001.

Subscription rates: Subscriptions run for a full calendar year. Prices are given per volume.
Personal subscription:
Subscription + postage and handling
CHF 124.35 + CHF 18.25 Europe
CHF 124.35 + CHF 27.20 Overseas
USD 95.00 + USD 18.25
+ online subscription per volume:
CHF 39.– / USD 30.00
(Must be in the name of, billed to, and paid by an individual. Order must be marked 'personal subscription'.)
Institutional subscription:
Subscription + postage and handling
CHF 852.– + CHF 22.80 Europe
CHF 852.– + CHF 34.– Overseas
USD 655.00 + USD 22.80
+ online subscription per volume:
CHF 58.– / USD 45.00
Airmail postage: CHF 24.–, USD 20.00.
(Extra per volume.)
Discount subscription prices:
Please enquire about reduced rates for residents.

Microforms: Please direct all enquiries and orders to:
University Microfilms Inc.
300 North Zeeb Road, P.O. Box 1346
Ann Arbor, MI 48106-1346 (USA)

Subscription orders: Orders can be placed at agencies, bookstores, directly with the
Publisher S. Karger AG, P.O. Box,
CH–4009 Basel (Switzerland)
or with any of the following distributors:
Deutschland: S. Karger GmbH, Postfach
D–79095 Freiburg
France: Librairie Luginbühl
36, bd de Latour-Maubourg, F–75007 Paris
Great Britain, Ireland: S. Karger Publishers
58 Grove Hill Road
Tunbridge Wells, Kent TN1 1SP, UK
USA: S. Karger Publishers, Inc.
26 West Avon Road, P.O. Box 529
Farmington, CT 06085, USA
India, Bangladesh, Sri Lanka:
Panther Publishers Private Ltd.
39, 6th Cross
Wilson Gardens
Bangalore 560 027, India
Japan: Katakura Libri, Inc.
2F, Marushima Bldg, 4-6-17, Yushima,
Bunkyo-ku, Tokyo 113-0034, Japan

Change of address: Both old and new address should be sent to the subscription source.

Single issues: Information can be obtained through the Publisher.

Advertising: Correspondence and rate requests should be addressed to the Publisher.

Bibliographic indices: This journal is regularly listed in bibliographic services, including *Current Contents*®.

Book Reviews: Books are accepted for review by special agreement.

Copying: This journal has been registered with the Copyright Clearance Center (CCC), as indicated by the code appearing on the first page of each article. For readers in the US, this code signals consent for copying of articles for personal or internal use, or for the personal or internal use of specific clients, provided that the stated fee is paid per copy directly to
Copyright Clearance Center Inc.
222 Rosewood Drive
Danvers, MA 01923 (USA).
A copy of the first page of the article must accompany payment. Consent does not extend to copying for general distribution, for promotion, for creating new works, or for resale. In these cases, specific written permission must be obtained from the copyright owner,
S. Karger AG, P.O. Box,
CH–4009 Basel (Switzerland).

KARGER

Fax + 41 61 306 12 34
E-Mail karger@karger.ch
www.karger.com

The Journal Home Page is available at:
www.karger.com/journals/ddi

Digestive Diseases

Functional Gastrointestinal Disorders

Editor

Peter Malfertheiner, Magdeburg

12 figures, 13 tables, 2001

KARGER

Basel · Freiburg · Paris · London · New York · New Delhi · Bangkok · Singapore · Tokyo · Sydney

S. Karger
Medical and Scientific Publishers
Basel · Freiburg · Paris · London
New York · New Delhi · Bangkok
Singapore · Tokyo · Sydney

Drug Dosage
The authors and the publisher have exerted every effort to ensure that drug selection and dosage set forth in this text are in accord with current recommendations and practice at the time of publication. However, in view of ongoing research, changes in government regulations, and the constant flow of information relating to drug therapy and drug reactions, the reader is urged to check the package insert for each drug for any change in indications and dosage and for added warnings and precautions. This is particularly important when the recommended agent is a new and/or infrequently employed drug.

P.O. Box, CH–4009 Basel (Switzerland)
Printed in Switzerland on acid-free paper by
Reinhardt Druck, Basel
ISBN 3–8055–7257–3

KARGER

Fax + 41 61 306 12 34
E-Mail karger@karger.ch
www.karger.com

Vol. 19, No. 3, 2001

Digestive Diseases

Contents

KARGER

Fax + 41 61 306 12 34
E-Mail karger@karger.ch
www.karger.com

Access to full text and tables of contents, including tentative ones for forthcoming issues:
www.karger.com/journals/ddi/ddi_bk.htm

Digestive Diseases

Dig Dis 2001;19:188

Editorial

The clinical management of functional disorders of the digestive system has become a major challenge at the level of primary care medicine and in specialist settings. Still now in clinical reality, we are often unable to provide patients a sufficient explanation of the cause of their symptoms and, even more, we often have great difficulties to achieve complete symptom relief with the available therapies. We are often left with the still important mission to reassure the patient that no organic disease is the cause of his suffering.

However, there is some progress and for subsets of patients with functional gastrointestinal disorders we can offer successful treatment by selecting the adequate therapeutic principle. The aim of this issue dedicated to the functional disorders of the upper and lower digestive tract is to provide an update on current facts and trends in this field including clinical assessment and novel diagnostic technologies. The currently available therapy principles as well as those that are in prospect are presented critically. This issue will also stimulate our awareness of the complexicity of the visceral sensory network involved in this heterogeneous disease complex as well as present the current aspects of functional abnormalities associated with abdominal symptoms. There is hope and promise that from the understanding of basic mechanisms new treatment principles will be derived.

Peter Malfertheiner

KARGER

Fax + 41 61 306 12 34
E-Mail karger@karger.ch
www.karger.com

0257–2753/01/0193–0188$17.50/0

Accessible online at:
www.karger.com/journals/ddi

Review Article

Digestive Diseases

Dig Dis 2001;19:189–194

Epidemiological Trends of Functional Gastrointestinal Disorders

J.M. Gschossmann S. Haag G. Holtmann

Department of Gastroenterology and Hepatology, University of Essen, Germany

Key Words

Functional gastrointestinal disorders · Epidemiology · Symptoms

Abstract

Functional gastrointestinal disorders are highly prevalent in the population and in primary and secondary care centers. Most likely they have been highly prevalent for centuries but in the past the lack of appropriate diagnostic measures did not enable the precise exclusion of structural causes of symptoms. In recent decades the prevalence rates of *Helicobacter pylori* has clearly decreased. As a result the incidence of *H. pylori*-related structural diseases in the upper gut decreased. Thus the relative proportion of functional gastrointestinal disorders has increased and may result in the overall impression that the prevalence of functional gastrointestinal disorders has increased. Thus, the available data do not provide evidence that the prevalence of these disorders has changed in recent decades.

Introduction

The primary target of this review is to identify potential time-dependent changes in the prevalence of functional gastrointestinal disorders. However, before an attempt to answer this question can be made, a critical review of the definitions of these disorders is needed and definitions used in various clinical trials need to be compared. Functional disorders of the gastrointestinal tract are characterized by symptoms referred to the gastrointestinal tract without evidence for structural or biochemical abnormalities that explain these symptoms. In recent years, interest has started focusing on functional gastrointestinal disorders since the widespread use of diagnostic procedures such as endoscopy, sonography and others revealed that underlying structural lesions are found only in approximately 50% of patients referred for evaluation of abdominal symptoms [1]. This increase in the clinical recognition is reflected by a marked increase in publications in this field during recent decades (fig. 1a, b).

Patients with functional gastrointestinal disorders present with a wide spectrum of symptoms. Consensus-based, they are categorized in a number of different disorders [2]. The two major single entities among functional disorders of the gut are functional dyspepsia and irritable bowel syndrome. Patients with functional dyspepsia characteristically localize the symptoms in the upper abdomen. Functional gastrointestinal disturbances which are localized in the lower abdomen are summarized as irritable bowel syndrome.

KARGER

Fax + 41 61 306 12 34
E-Mail karger@karger.ch
www.karger.com

0257–2753/01/0193–0189$17.50/0

Accessible online at:
www.karger.com/journals/ddi

Prof. Dr. med. Gerald Holtmann
Division of Internal Medicine
Department of Gastroenterology and Hepatology, University of Essen
Hufelandstrasse 55, D–45122 Essen (Germany)
Tel. +49 201 723 3618, Fax +49 201 723 5970, E-Mail g.holtmann@uni-essen.de

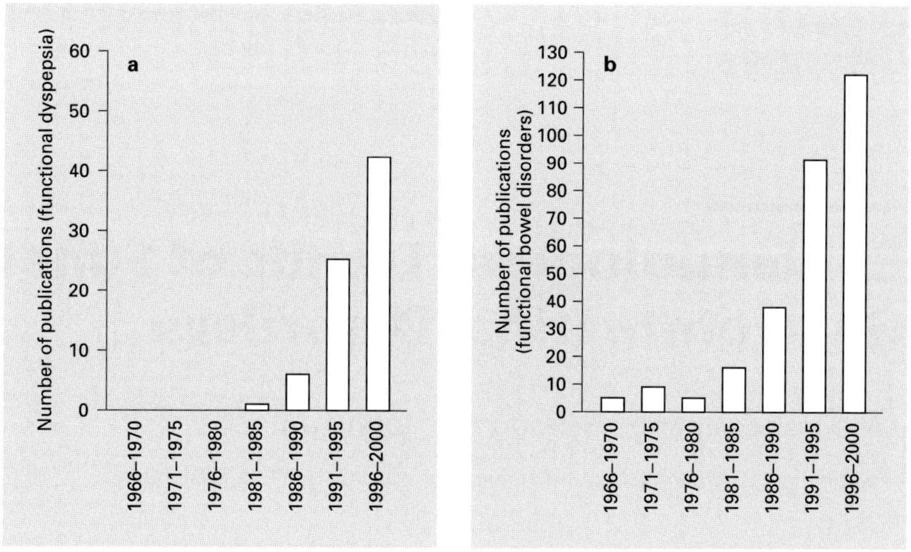

Fig. 1. Number of scientific publications cited in Medline for functional dyspepsia (**a**) and irritable bowel syndrome (**b**).

Table 1. A collection of dyspepsia definitions: there is general agreement that the diagnosis of functional dyspepsia requires to rule out a structural or biochemical abnormality [modified from 48]

Group	Year	Definition of dyspepsia
Rhind and Watson [23]	1968	Epigastric discomfort after meals, fullness so that tight clothing is loosened, eructation with temporary relief, and regurgitation of sour fluid into the mouth, with heartburn 'flatulent dyspepsia'
Crean et al. [22]	1982	Any form of episodic or persistent abdominal discomfort or other symptom referable to the alimentary tract, except jaundice and gastrointestinal bleeding are excluded
Thompson [24]	1984	Chronic, recurrent, often meal-related epigastric discomfort
Lagarde and Spiro [25]	1984	Intermittent upper abdominal pain or discomfort
Talley and Piper [26]	1985	Intermittent or continuous pain, discomfort, or nausea referable to the upper alimentary tract; present for a month or more; is not precipitated by exertion and relieved by rest; not associated with jaundice, bleeding, or dysphagia
Nyrén et al. [27]	1987	Key symptoms are epigastric pain or discomfort, absence of irritable bowel symptoms and organic disease 'epigastric distress syndrome'
Talley and Phillips [28]	1988	Chronic or recurrent upper abdominal pain or nausea that may or may not be related to meals and a duration of at least 3 months
Colin-Jones et al. [29]	1988	Upper abdominal or retrosternal pain, discomfort, heartburn, nausea, vomiting, or other symptom considered to be referable to the proximal alimentary tract
Barbara et al. [30]	1989	Episodic or persistent abdominal symptoms, often related to feeding, that patients or physicians believe to be due to disorders of the proximal portion of the digestive tract
Heading [31]	1991	Episodic or persistent abdominal symptoms that include abdominal pain or discomfort; the term 'dyspepsia' is not applied to patients whose symptoms are thought to be arising from outside the proximal gastrointestinal tract
Working Team, Talley et al. [32]	1991	Persistent or recurrent abdominal pain or abdominal discomfort centered in the upper abdomen

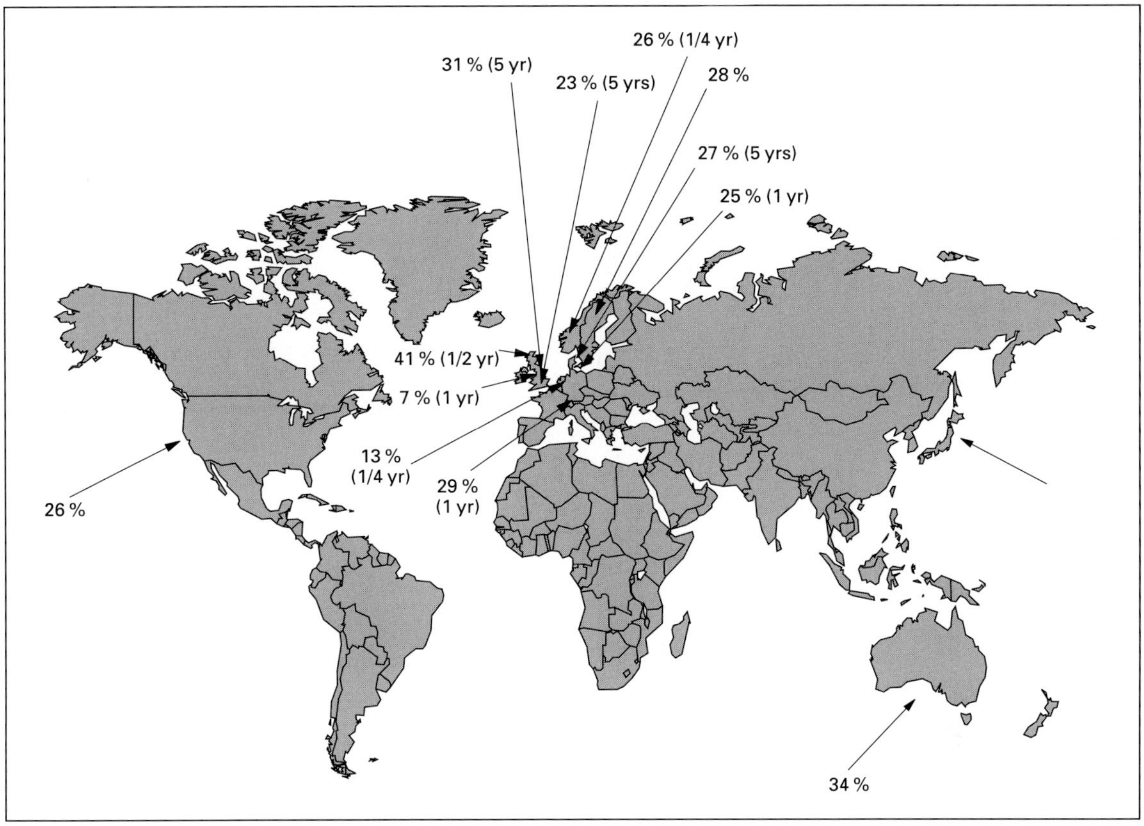

Fig. 2. Prevalence of dyspeptic symptoms and peptic ulcers in different populations [3, 4, 6–18] (1-year prevalence rates if not otherwise stated).

Prevalence and Incidence of Functional Gastrointestinal Disorders in the Population

Both dyspepsia and irritable bowel syndrome represent a set of symptoms rather than a precisely defined condition. Population-based studies from various geographic regions observed for dyspepsia prevalence rates range from 7 to 41%, while most population-based studies yield prevalence rates from 20 to 30% [3] (fig. 2). Similarly, the irritable bowel syndrome represents a widespread syndrome and accounts for one of the most frequent diseases worldwide. Epidemiological studies in different countries and continents generated prevalence rates between 6 and 25% [3–21].

Prevalence rates are not correlated ($r < 0.4$, $p > 0.5$) with the year of publication suggesting that there is no clear time trend (fig. 3). However, the variability of prevalence rates is remarkable. This variability of prevalence may partly reflect differences in the 'true' prevalence of dyspepsia and irritable bowel syndrome. However, numerous definitions for dyspepsia (and consequently for

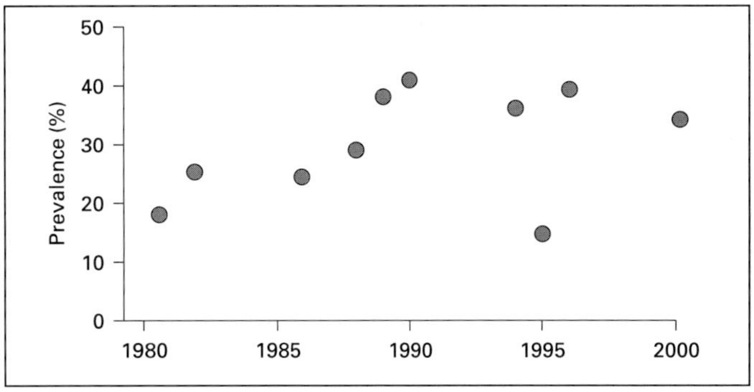

Fig. 3. Lack of an association between the year of publication and prevalence rates of dyspepsia (1-year rate) in population-based studies ($r < 0.4$, $p > 0.2$).

functional dyspepsia) have been proposed in the literature [22–32]. These authors suggested definitions that were focused on quite different aspects of the spectrum of upper abdominal symptoms (table 1). Several authors have restricted dyspepsia to meal-related symptoms [24,

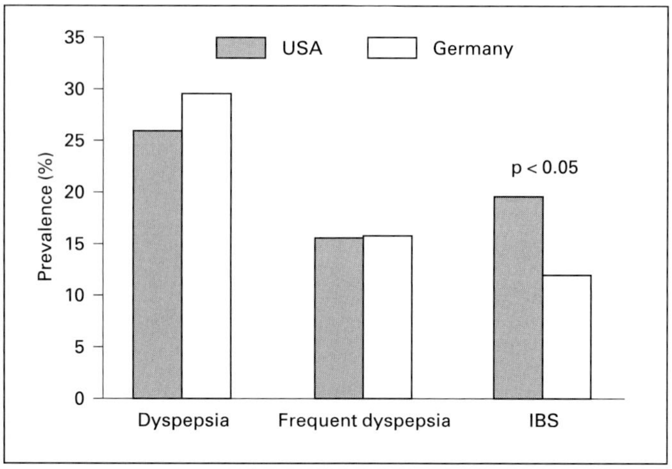

Fig. 4. Prevalence rates for dyspepsia in two trials from different regions utilizing the same methodology for the assessment of symptoms [3].

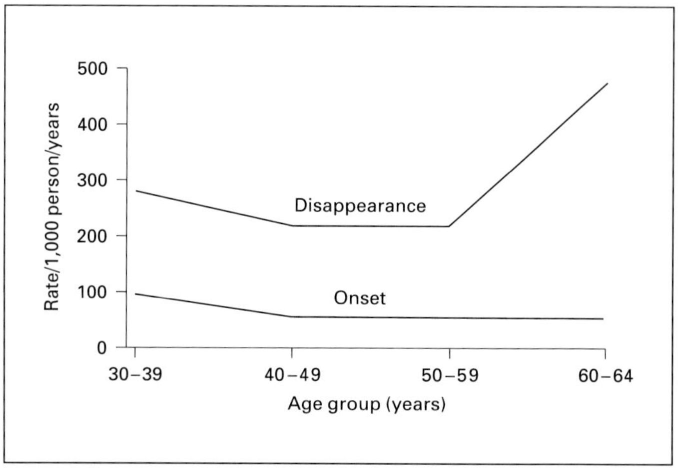

Fig. 5. Onset and disappearance of dyspepsia [36].

33]. In contrast, conditions such as peptic ulcer disease, which is considered to be a classical cause of dyspepsia, do not cause symptoms that are exclusively confined to the pre- or postprandial period [34, 35]. Thus there is now general agreement that dyspepsia is not restricted to meal-related symptoms.

Besides differences in definitions, several other issues have to be taken into account. It is important to emphasize that most population-based studies assessed subjects with 'undiagnosed' dyspepsia or irritable bowel syndrome. Thus, a considerable but not precisely defined proportion of subjects with structural lesions will be included in these studies. The proportion of subjects with structural lesions as a cause of symptoms might be variable. For example, the prevalence of the infection with *Helicobacter pylori* – that can be considered to be a conditio sine qua non for peptic ulcers – is highly variable in different populations. In addition, *H. pylori* prevalence rates have decreased in recent decades with a decrease of associated peptic ulcers. Thus, the variability of *H. pylori* prevalence rates may contribute to the reported variability of dyspepsia. Other important factors, however, are criteria and methodology for the assessment of symptoms. Technically, prevalence of dyspepsia or irritable bowel syndrome is defined as the proportion of subjects reporting a set of symptoms at a specific day. Hence, symptoms may occur on a given day and disappear the next; the prevalence of dyspepsia or irritable bowel syndrome on a given day is not a useful measure. Indeed most investigators assessed the 1-year prevalence. In addition, the frequency of symptom occurrence has been included by some investigators to identify subjects with more severe symptoms and to exclude subjects with only occasional symptom manifestation.

The assumption that the reported variability of functional bowel disorders is caused by methodological issues is supported by the results of two trials from different regions utilizing the same methodology for the assessment of symptoms. Both studies yielded very similar prevalence rates for dyspepsia [3, 4] (fig. 4) while the prevalence of irritable bowel syndrome was slightly higher in the USA.

While the prevalence of these disorders has been extensively studied, little data are available on the incidence of these disorders. However, one population-based study from Olmsted County observed during a 12- to 20-month follow-up new symptoms that were compatible with functional abdominal symptoms in approximately 9% of the study population, while the same number of subjects who initially reported symptoms became symptom-free [36] (fig. 5). In another study the calculated 3-month incidence of dyspepsia for previously asymptomatic subjects was 0.8% (95% CI 0.0–1.6) [37].

Dyspepsia and Irritable Bowel Syndrome in Clinical Practice and Healthcare-Seeking Behavior

The proportion of subjects suffering from dyspepsia and irritable bowel syndrome seeking medical care is believed to be less than 50% [3, 4, 38–40]. Nevertheless, conservative estimates suggest that these disorders account for 2–5% of all consultations in general practice; up to one-third of these patients may eventually be referred to a gastroenterologist [41]. One important issue is the motivation for seeking medical care, another the intensity of symptoms. Subjects with intense abdominal (and extraintestinal) symptoms are more likely to seek medical attention [4]. In addition, psychological distress may also affect the utilization of healthcare services [42]. Indeed patients with functional dyspepsia score higher on scales measuring neuroticism and anxiety [43, 44]. Similar to irritable bowel syndrome [42], these psychological features might be characteristic for subjects that seek medical attention (even at tertiary referral centers).

An important issue is the chronicity of functional symptoms. Longitudinal studies have shown a remarkable stability of the prevalence over time [36, 37, 45, 46]. This is the result of subjects with new onset dyspepsia and subjects who do not report symptom recurrence. Interestingly, 30% of patients treated for dyspepsia have symptom resolution followed for 1 year [47]. On the other hand, disappearance of dyspepsia does not equal absence of abdominal symptoms; in a Swedish study [37], 57% of patients had resolution of dyspeptic symptoms after 1 year. However, only 12% were without abdominal symptoms. The remaining suffered irritable bowel syndrome or reflux symptoms.

Conclusions

Functional gastrointestinal disorders are highly prevalent in the population and in primary and secondary care centers. They have most likely been highly prevalent for centuries but in the past the lack of appropriate diagnostic measures did not allow to precisely exclude structural causes of symptoms. In recent decades the prevalence rates of *H. pylori* has clearly decreased. As the result, the incidence of *H. pylori*-related structural diseases has decreased. Thus the relative proportion of functional gastrointestinal disorders has increased and may result in the overall impression that the prevalence of functional gastrointestinal disorders has increased.

Since appropriate cohort studies are lacking, prevalence rates from various studies must be used for the assessment of changes in the prevalence of functional gastrointestinal disorders. Unfortunately, definitions for these disorders have been steadily changed. This makes it very difficult or virtually impossible to compare prevalence rates from different time periods or geographic regions. Thus, the available data do not provide evidence that the prevalence of these disorders has changed.

References

1 Talley NJ, Silverstein MD, Agréus L, Nyrén O, Sonnenberg A, Holtmann G: Evaluation of dyspepsia. Gastroenterology 1998;114:582–595.

2 Talley NJ, Stanghellini V, Heading RC, Koch KL, Malagelada JR, Tytgat GN: Functional gastroduodenal disorders. Gut 1999;45(suppl 2):II37–II42.

3 Talley NJ, Zinsmeister AR, Schleck CD, Melton LJI: Dyspepsia and dyspepsia subgroups: A population-based study. Gastroenterology 1992;102:1259–1268.

4 Holtmann G, Goebell H, Talley NJ: Dyspepsia in consulters and non-consulters: Prevalence, health-care seeking behaviour and risk factors. Eur J Gastroenterol Hepatol 1994;6:917–924.

5 Schlemper R, Van der Werf SDJ, Vandenbroucke JP, Biemond I, Lamers CBHW: Peptic ulcer, non-ulcer dyspepsia and irritable bowel syndrome in The Netherlands and Japan. Scand J Gastroenterol Suppl 1993;200:33–41.

6 Doll R, Jones FA, Buckatzsch MM: Occupational factors in the aetiology of gastric and duodenal ulcers with an estimate of their incidence in the general population. Med Res Counc Spec Rep Ser

7 Weir RD, Backett EM: Studies of the epidemiology of peptic ulcer in a rural community: Prevalence and natural history of dyspepsia and peptic ulcer. Gut 1968;9:75–83.

8 Banke L: Ulcumygdommers epidemiologi. Copenhagen, FADL Publishers, 1975.

9 Thompson WG, Heaton KW: Functional bowel disorders in apparently healthy people. Gastroenterology 1980;79:283–288.

10 Hollnagel H, Norrelund N, Larsen S: Marvetarmsymptomer blandt 40-arige i Glostrup: en epidemiologisk undersogelse. Ugeskr Laeger 1982;144:267–273.

11 Shirlow MJ, Mathers CD: A study of caffeine consumption and symptoms: Indigestion, palpitations, tremor, headache, and insomnia. Int J Epidemiol 1985;14:239–248.

12 Tibblin G: Introduction to the epidemiology of dyspepsia. Scand J Gastroenterol Suppl 1985; 109:29–33.

13 Johnsen R, Straume B, Forde OH: Peptic ulcer and non-ulcer dyspepsia – A disease and a disorder. Scand J Prim Health Care 1988;6:239–243.

14 Jones RH, Lydeard SE, Hobbs FDR, Kenkre JE, Williams EI, Jones SJ, Pepper JA, Dunwoodie WMB, Bottomey JM: Dyspepsia in England and Scotland. Gut 1990;31:401–405.

15 Harrison JD, Morris DL: Dyspepsia in coalminers and the general population: A comparative study. Br J Ind Med 1989;46:428–429.

16 Bernersen B, Johnsen R, Straume B, Burhol PG, Jenssen TG, Stakkevold PA: Towards a true prevalence of peptic ulcer: The Sorreisa gastrointestinal disorder study. Gut 1990;31: 989–992.

17 Schlemper RJ, Van der Werf SDJ, Vandenbroucke JP, Biemond I, Lamers CBHW: Nonulcer dyspepsia in a Dutch working population and *Helicobacter pylori*: Ulcer history as an explanation of an apparent association. Arch Intern Med 1995;155:82–87.

18 Jones R, Lydeard S: Prevalence of symptoms of dyspepsia in the community. BMJ 1989;298: 30–32.

19 Haag S, Holtmann G, Neufang-Huber J, Gschossmann J, Gerken G, Talley NJ: Is there a link between the pattern of functional abdominal symptoms and disturbances of gastric emptying or the response to a nutrient challenge? Gastroenterology 2000;118.

20 Agreus L, Svardsudd K, Nyren O, Tibblin G: Irritable bowel syndrome and dyspepsia in the general population: Overlap and lack of stability over time. Gastroenterology 1995;109:671–680.
21 Giacosa A, Sukkar SG, Gogioso L: Dyspepsia among young conscripts: Correlations with psychoemotional state and eating habits. J R Army Med Corps 1987;133:59–62.
22 Crean GP, et al: Ulcer-like dyspepsia. Scand J Gastroenterol 1982;17(suppl 79):9–15.
23 Rhind JA, Watson L: Gall stone dyspepsia. BMJ 1968;1:32.
24 Thompson WG: Nonulcer dyspepsia. Can Med Assoc J 1984;130:565–569.
25 Lagarde SP, Spiro HM: Non-ulcer dyspepsia. Clin Gastroenterol 1984;13:437–446.
26 Talley NJ, Piper DW: The association between non-ulcer dyspepsia and other gastrointestinal disorders. Scand J Gastroenterol 1985;20:896–900.
27 Nyrén O, Adami HO, Gustavsson S, Lindgren PG, Loof L, Nyberg A: The 'epigastric distress syndrome'. A possible disease entity identified by history and endoscopy in patients with nonulcer dyspepsia. J Clin Gastroenterol 1987;9:303–309.
28 Talley NJ, Phillips SF: Non-ulcer dyspepsia: Potential causes and pathophysiology. Ann Intern Med 1988;108:865–879.
29 Colin-Jones DG, Bloom B, Bodemar G, Crean G, Freston J, Gugler R, Malagelada J, Nyrén O, Petersen H, Piper D: Management of dyspepsia: Report of a working party. Lancet 1988; i:576–579.
30 Barbara L, Camilleri M, Corinaldesi R, Crean GP, Heading RC, Johnson AG, Malagelada JR, Stanghellini V, Wienbeck M: Definition and investigation of dyspepsia. Consensus of an international ad hoc working party. Dig Dis Sci 1989;34:1272–1276.
31 Heading RC: Definitions of dyspepsia. Scand J Gastroenterol Suppl 1991;182:1–6.
32 Talley NJCJ, Koch KL, Koch M, Nyrén O, Stanghellini V: Functional dyspepsia: A classification with guidelines for diagnosis and management. Gastroenterol Int 1991;4:145–160.
33 Malagelada JR, Stanghellini V: Manometric evaluation of functional upper gut symptoms. Gastroenterology 1985;88:1223–1231.
34 Crean GP, Holden RJ, Knill-Jones RP, Beattie AD, James WB, Marjoribanks FM, Spiegelhalter DJ: A database on dyspepsia. Gut 1994; 35:191–202.
35 Earlam RJ: Endoscopic and histological findings in subjects with dyspepsia. BMJ 1991;302: 1153.
36 Talley NJ, Weaver AL, Zinsmeister AR, Melton LJI: Onset and disappearance of gastrointestinal symptoms and functional gastrointestinal disorders. Am J Epidemiol 1992;136:165–177.
37 Agreus L, Svärdsudd K, Nyren O, Tibblin G: Irritable bowel syndrome and dyspepsia in the general population: Overlap and lack of stability over time. Gastroenterology 1995;109:671–680.
38 Gaburri M, Bassotti G, Bacci G, Cinti A, Bosso R, Ceccarelli P, Paolocci N, Pelli MA, Morelli A: Functional gut disorders and health care seeking behavior in an Italian non-patient population. Recent Prog Med 1989;80:241–244.
39 Sandler RS, Drossman DA, Nathan HP, McKee DC: Symptom complaints and health care seeking behavior in subjects with bowel dysfunction. Gastroenterology 1984;87:314–318.
40 Zuckerman MJ, Guerra LG, Drossman DA, Foland JA, Gregory GG: Health-care-seeking behaviors related to bowel complaints: Hispanics versus non-Hispanic whites. Dig Dis Sci 1996;41:77–82.
41 Knill-Jones RP: Geographical differences in the prevalence of dyspepsia. Scand J Gastroenterol 1991;26(suppl 182):17–24.
42 Whitehead WE, Bosmajian L, Zorderman AB, Costa PT, Schuster MM: Symptoms of psychologic distress associated with irritable bowel syndrome. Comparison of community and medical clinic samples. Gastroenterology 1988; 95:709–714.
43 Wilson KC, Whiteoak R, Dewey M, Watson JP: Aspects of personality of soldiers presenting to an endoscopy clinic. J Psychosom Res 1989; 33:85–91.
44 Haug TT, Svebak S, Hausken T, Wilhelmsen I, Berstad A, Ursin H: Low vagal activity as mediating mechanism for the relationship between personality factors and gastric symptoms in functional dyspepsia. Psychosom Med 1994; 56:181–186.
45 Jones R, Lydeard S: Dyspepsia in the community: A follow-up study. Br J Clin Pract 1992; 46:95–97.
46 Kay L, Jorgensen T: Epidemiology of upper dyspepsia in a random population. Scand J Gastroenterol 1994;29:1–6.
47 Talley NJ, McNeil D, Hayden A, Colreavy C, Piper DW: Prognosis of chronic unexplained dyspepsia. A prospective study of potential predictor variables in patients with endoscopically diagnosed nonulcer dyspepsia. Gastroenterology 1987;92:1060–1066.
48 Holtmann G, Stanghellini V, Talley NJ: Nomenclature of dyspepsia, dyspepsia subgroups and functional dyspepsia: Clarifying the concepts. Baillières Clin Gastroenterol 1998;12: 417–433.

Review Article

Digestive Diseases

Dig Dis 2001;19:195–200

Targeting the Abnormalities of Gastroduodenal Functions in Functional Dyspepsia

J. Enrique Domínguez-Muñoz

Department of Gastroenterology, University Hospital of Santiago de Compostela, Spain

Key Words
Acid secretion · Gastrointestinal motility · Gastric emptying · Visceral sensitivity · *Helicobacter pylori* · Bacterial overgrowth

Abstract
The current definition of functional dyspepsia changes the previous concept of absence of organic disease to the presence of a functional alteration of the upper gastrointestinal tract. From a theoretical point of view, the alteration of any major gastrointestinal function may induce dyspeptic symptoms. However, both asymptomatic subjects with some gastrointestinal functional alteration and dyspeptic patients without a demonstrable dysfunction are not unusual. This may be explained at least in part by the more recent concept of visceral sensitivity. The potential role of acid secretion in the pathogenesis of functional dyspepsia as well as the positive effect of antisecretory drugs in a proportion of patients may be based on an increased gastric acid secretion and duodenal acid overload, a hypersensitivity to acid and/or the development of acid-mediated gastrointestinal motor abnormalities. *Helicobacter pylori* infection may play a role in this context. Both interdigestive and postprandial gastrointestinal motility, mainly a delayed gastric emptying and an altered intragastric distribution of nutrients, have been described to be disturbed in up to half of the patients with functional dyspepsia. This may also be an explanation for the high frequency of intestinal bacterial overgrowth in these patients. Most probably, visceral hypersensitivity should be present for motor alterations to induce symptoms. This is the basis for future development of new drugs in the management of this functional syndrome. The role of *H. pylori* in the pathogenesis of functional dyspepsia is a matter of discussion, but a proportion of patients benefit from eradication therapy and, therefore this therapeutic approach should be taken into account.

The definition of dyspepsia of non-organic origin has changed in the last years. The previous negative concept of 'non-ulcer dyspepsia', indicating the absence of an organic disease to explain the symptoms, has moved to a positive one, the 'functional dyspepsia' concept which reinforces the presence of a functional alteration in the stomach and/or proximal small intestine as the origin of the abdominal symptomatology.

The acid secretion and the grinding and emptying of nutrients are the main functions of the stomach. On the

KARGER

Fax + 41 61 306 12 34
E-Mail karger@karger.ch
www.karger.com

0257–2753/01/0193–0195$17.50/0

Accessible online at:
www.karger.com/journals/ddi

J. Enrique Domínguez-Muñoz, MD
Department of Gastroenterology
University Hospital, C/Choupana, s/n
E-15706-Santiago de Compostela (Spain)
Tel. +34 981 950 070, Fax +34 981 951 378, E-Mail jdominguezm@medynet.com

other hand, the small intestine has, together with digestive and absorptive functions, an important motor activity both in the postprandial as well as in the interdigestive state. Both gastric and intestinal functions are coordinated by different reflexes, in which neural connections and hormone release are involved. From a theoretical point of view, the alteration of any of these functions may originate abdominal symptoms, either directly or indirectly, through the development of several disturbances like intestinal bacterial overgrowth. This has been the basis of the ongoing concept of functional dyspepsia over the last years. However, these functional alterations in the proximal gastrointestinal tract have been described in asymptomatic subjects and, in addition, patients with dyspeptic symptoms in whom no functional abnormality is found are not uncommon.

More recently, visceral sensitivity has centered the attempts of researchers to explain dyspeptic symptoms. According to this concept, subjects with functional dyspepsia could be able to perceive as abdominal pain or discomfort either physiological visceral stimuli (i.e. gastrointestinal distension or contraction) or gastrointestinal functional alterations that are normally not perceived by the majority of subjects. This would explain the presence of symptoms in those dyspeptic subjects with no demonstrable gastrointestinal functional alteration as well as the absence of symptoms in subjects with functional disturbances of the stomach or proximal small intestine. According to this concept, visceral hypersensitivity would be responsible for symptoms in some patients with dyspepsia, either with or without any demonstrable functional alteration, and a normal or even reduced visceral sensitivity would be present in asymptomatic subjects with gastrointestinal functional disturbances.

The present article aims to discuss the different abnormalities of gastroduodenal functions that have been involved in functional dyspepsia as well as the potential role of visceral hypersensitivity in this disease. This is the basis for an adequate diagnostic and therapeutic approach to functional dyspepsia.

Targeting the Abnormalities of Gastric Acid Secretion

The majority of clinical studies on functional dyspepsia have failed to find a significant association between the occurrence of the syndrome and any gastrointestinal functional alteration. This is at least in part due to the different functional disturbances that can be responsible for a similar symptomatology and that these disturbances may also be present in asymptomatic controls. In this way, the probability that the etiological factor under evaluation is significantly more frequent in patients than in controls is not high.

The potential role of the abnormalities of gastric acid secretion is not an exception to this rule. From a theoretical point of view, an increased acid secretion and duodenal acid overload could be responsible for dyspepsia in patients with predominant fasting abdominal pain (ulcer-like symptomatology) in whom the presence of ulcer cannot be demonstrated. This has been, however, an inconsistent finding in different clinical studies [1]. In general, basal gastric acid secretion in patients with functional dyspepsia has been reported to be similar to that in asymptomatic controls but significantly lower than that in patients with duodenal ulcer [2, 3]. Similar results have been found with regard to stimulated gastric acid secretion [3]. In addition, no difference in gastric acid secretion, either basal or stimulated, seems to exist between different groups of dyspeptic patients according to the major symptom [3].

Studies on the correlation between gastric acid secretion and functional dyspepsia have consistently ignored the role of *Helicobacter pylori* infection. However, *H. pylori* is the major factor modifying gastric acid secretion. About 40–50% of dyspeptic patients are not infected by *H. pylori* and, as a consequence, gastric acid secretion in these patients is mostly normal. Among the remaining 50–60% of patients with functional dyspepsia and *H. pylori* infection, some will have an antrum-predominant chronic gastritis and therefore an increased gastric acid secretion, and the remaining ones will develop a pangastritis or corpus-predominant gastritis that is frequently associated with a reduced gastric acid secretion. All these patients suffer from dyspeptic symptoms but only some of them have an increased gastric acid secretion. This is actually related to the presence of *H. pylori* infection and symptoms in these patients may be secondary to other *H. pylori*-related abnormalities and not only to acid.

A second possibility is that at least some dyspeptic patients are hypersensitive to acid. In fact, patients with functional dyspepsia and not asymptomatic controls refer frequently pain after duodenal instillation of acid [4, 5]. Furthermore, instillation of acid within the duodenal bulb triggers gastrointestinal motor abnormalities in dyspeptic patients but not in control subjects [5]. These motor abnormalities (abnormal clearance of acid, reduced frequency and duration of interdigestive gastrointestinal motor migration complexes) are associated with the development of dyspeptic symptoms and revert by inhibiting gastric acid secretion [5, 6].

Either an abnormally high gastric acid secretion and/or a hypersensitivity to acid and/or the development of acid-mediated gastrointestinal motor abnormalities may explain, together with the consistent placebo effect in these patients, the positive therapeutic response to gastric acid inhibition in patients with functional dyspepsia that is repeatedly observed in clinical routine and has also been reported in clinical studies [7].

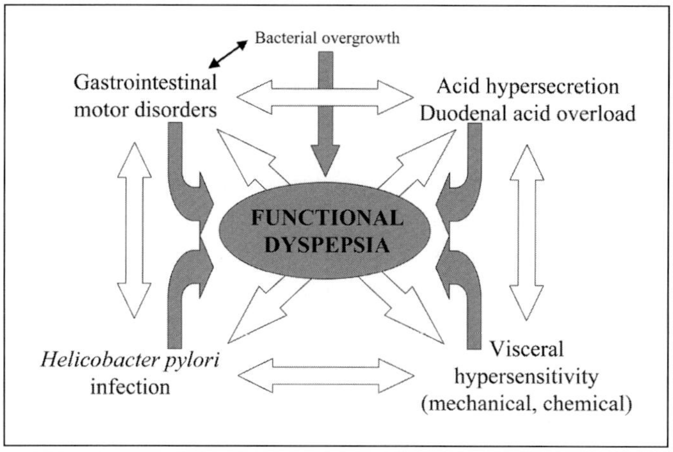

Fig. 1. Abnormalities of gastrointestinal function involved in the pathogenesis of functional dyspepsia and interrelationship among them.

Targeting the Abnormalities of Gastrointestinal Motility

Since symptoms in functional dyspepsia are characterized by pain or discomfort, fullness, abdominal distension and/or nausea that frequently are related to meal ingestion, motility disorders mainly of the stomach have classically been considered as a major disturbance in these patients. In addition to the general problems discussed above with regard to clinical studies in dyspepsia, some other limitations exist to demonstrate the relationship between motor disorders of the proximal gastrointestinal tract and functional dyspepsia. One of the major limitations relies on the methodological difficulties to accurately evaluate motor function of the gastrointestinal tract. Furthermore, and as discussed above, the heterogeneity of functional dyspepsia makes difficult to demonstrate a correlation between motor disturbances and symptoms and, together with the important placebo effect of any therapeutic approach in these patients, this limits the quantification of the real effect of any prokinetic therapy.

Both interdigestive and postprandial gastric and intestinal motility have been described to be altered in around half of the patients with functional dyspepsia. During the interdigestive state, the most frequent abnormality described regards the origin, frequency and amplitude of phase III of the motor migrating complex (MMC) [8–10]. In this sense in patients with functional dyspepsia, phase III of the motor migrating complex is less frequent, less frequently originates from the stomach and the wave amplitude is lower than in controls. Although these findings are not consistently observed in patients with functional dyspepsia and could not be confirmed by other authors [11, 12], the presence of these motor alterations at least partially explain the greater frequency of bacterial overgrowth found in these patients [13]. Furthermore, and making more complicated the interrelationship of different etiopathogenic factors in the origin of functional dyspepsia, bacterial overgrowth in the proximal intestine in these patients is more frequent in the presence of *H. pylori* [13]. Treatment of bacterial overgrowth is associated with a significant clinical improvement but both bacterial overgrowth and symptoms relapse some weeks thereafter [13]. This indicates that both are secondary events, probably to primary motor abnormalities that may in some cases be related to the presence of *H. pylori* infection with some role for the resulting acid secretion abnormality (fig. 1).

In the postprandial state, functional dyspepsia is frequently associated with either a decreased contractile capacity of the antrum, a slow gastric emptying of solids and/or an abnormal intragastric distribution of nutrients [9, 14–16]. Postprandial gastric function is therefore altered in patients with functional dyspepsia and this can induce symptoms in some of them. Physiologically, solid nutrients are stored within the proximal stomach (fundus and proximal body) just after being ingested. This is possible because of the relaxation of the proximal stomach in response to gastro-gastric and duodeno-gastric reflexes mediated by nutrients. The consequence of this relaxation is the distension of the proximal stomach without increasing the intraluminal pressure and thus allowing the asymptomatic accommodation of the nutrients. As the amount of nutrients in the antrum and duodenum decreases, the tone of the proximal stomach increases and part of the nutrients are transported to the distal stomach (distal body and antrum). There, the solid particles are ground up to a diameter of <2 mm to be able to pass through the pylorus into the duodenum. Any of the different steps of this complex motor function of the stomach, which is regulated by intricate neural and hormonal reflexes, may be altered in functional dyspepsia and may lead in some patients to an abnormally delayed gastric emptying. Thus, one of the most frequent findings in these patients is a limited accommodative capacity of the proximal stomach leading to the distal accumulation of the meal and distension of the antrum [15].

Despite the frequent presence of the above-described motor alterations in patients with functional dyspepsia, this is not enough to explain symptoms in the vast majority of the patients. In fact, symptoms are usually not different in patients with and without demonstrable motor abnormality and the experimental induction of these motor alterations in humans does not induce symptoms [12]. Most probably, visceral hypersensitivity plays a key role in the perception of gastrointestinal motor alterations as dyspeptic symptoms.

From a therapeutic point of view, the knowledge of frequent gastrointestinal motor abnormalities in functional dyspepsia and the fact that symptoms frequently suggest the presence of these alterations have justified the routine use of prokinetic drugs in these patients. The scientific evidence in this respect is, however, conflicting. Different clinical studies have found that the positive effect of drugs like cisapride or domperidone on the motor function of the upper gastrointestinal tract is frequently but not consistently associated with a symptomatic improvement in patients with functional dyspepsia [17–19]. In fact, some studies have found that the prokinetic effect of cisapride is not accompanied by changes in visceral hypersensitivity [20, 21].

Targeting the Abnormalities of Visceral Hypersensitivity

Despite the potential presence of gastric motor abnormalities, the mechanical properties of the stomach in patients with functional dyspepsia are not disturbed. In fact, both compliance and distensibility, as evaluated by means of a gastric barostat, are similar in dyspeptic patients and in asymptomatic controls [22]. However, the sensitivity of the stomach to distension is abnormally high in patients with functional dyspepsia. According to that, these patients perceive as unpleasant or even painful pressures or volumes of distension that are unperceived or only lightly perceived by asymptomatic subjects or patients with organic dyspepsia [22–28], although this is not a constant finding in every dyspeptic patient [29].

Patients with functional dyspepsia are not generally hypersensitive. In fact, somatic sensitivity is consistently normal in these subjects [22]. A different aspect is whether visceral hypersensitivity is a generalized disorder that affects every segment of the gastrointestinal tract or whether this is a more specific disorder. The reported findings in this respect are controversial mainly due to different inclusion criteria of patients [25–27]. Visceral hypersensitivity is restricted to the stomach and occasionally also to the upper intestine in patients with pure functional dyspepsia. However, if functional dyspepsia is associated with irritable bowel syndrome, which is a frequent association, visceral hypersensitivity is more unspecific and affects almost any segment of the gastrointestinal tract [27].

The fact that visceral sensitivity in dyspeptic patients increases significantly after intraduodenal instillation of lipids [30] and that this intraduodenal lipid administration induces dyspeptic symptoms in these patients [31] may help to explain the relationship between symptoms and meals. Furthermore, this increase in visceral sensitivity is nutrient specific, since the administration of the same amount of calories as carbohydrates does not have the same effect as lipids [31]. This finding may be used therapeutically by dietary modifications.

The peripheral neural stimulation that is transmitted and modulated through the spinal cord to the brain is lastly responsible for dyspeptic symptoms like pain, fullness or nausea. In addition, this sensorial neural stimulation participates in the modulation through different local and central reflexes of other basic gastrointestinal functions like motility that, as mentioned above, is also involved in the origin of functional dyspepsia. Based on this, it makes sense to focus research for new therapeutic approaches in functional dyspepsia on drugs able either to suppress the primary afferent sensorial activity from the gut (i.e. analgesics like tricyclic antidepressants or opioid derivatives, and ion channels inhibitors) [32–34] or to inhibit selectively the neuronal sensorial hypersensitivity within the gastrointestinal tract. In this last process of sensorial neuronal activation within the myoenteric plexus, serotonin (5-HT) appears to play a major role [35]. Because of this, great efforts have been made over the last years to develop new drugs able to modulate both the extrinsic and intrinsic neural pathways mediated by serotonin, among them 5-HT_1 agonists and antagonists like 8-OH-DPAT or sumatriptan [36, 37], 5-HT_3 and 5-HT_4 antagonists like alosetron, granisetron or cilasetron [38], and 5-HT_4 agonists like tegaserod [39].

In summary, visceral hypersensitivity most probably plays a major role in the genesis of symptoms in functional dyspepsia, although this is surely not the only mechanism responsible for this syndrome. Over the last years, several mediators and receptors involved in visceral nociception, both within the myoenteric plexus and the central nervous system, have been described and are the objectives for the development of new drugs. Most of these drugs are still in the experimental animal research phase but probably in the near future they will change the therapeutic approach to patients with functional disorders.

The Role of *H. pylori* Infection

H. pylori infection is a generally recognized cause of functional alterations in the stomach. As mentioned above, *H. pylori*-related antrum-predominant gastritis is associated with an increased release of gastrin [40], mainly secondary to a reduced synthesis and release of somatostatin from antral D cells [41]. As a consequence, gastric acid secretion and duodenal acid load are increased in these patients [40, 42, 43]. This can be associated with changes in gastric motor function, although most studies on gastrointestinal motility have failed to demonstrate significant alterations in *H. pylori*-infected subjects [40, 44]. *H. pylori* infection also does not cause changes in visceral sensitivity, and gastric hypersensitivity to distension in dyspeptic patients is independent of the presence or absence of *H. pylori* [45]. As a result of all these data, it is debatable whether the *H. pylori*-induced changes in gastric physiology are able to be the origin of dyspeptic symptoms. Recently, we have confirmed that *H. pylori* infection is associated with hypergastrinemia and have shown for the first time that *H. pylori*-positive patients have an increased interdigestive pancreatic secretion without changes in interdigestive and postprandial gastrointestinal motility, release of pancreatic polypeptide and motilin [46]. Furthermore, coordination between gastrointestinal motility, pancreatic secretion and hormone release is not altered by *H. pylori* infection [46]. As a hypothesis, this pancreatic hypersecretion could be the origin of abdominal pain in some patients with impaired pancreatic outflow, which deserves further investigation.

From an epidemiological point of view, *H. pylori* infection is significantly more prevalent among dyspeptic patients than in asymptomatic subjects, with an absolute difference of 23% [47]. Furthermore, a Cochrane systematic review of the medical evidence demonstrated that *H. pylori* eradication is associated with the disappearance of or significant improvement in dyspeptic symptoms compared to a proton pump inhibitor at 6 or 12 months of follow-up [48]. This long-term positive effect of *H. pylori* eradication in functional dyspepsia has recently been demonstrated in a large multicenter study [49]. Therefore, although the etiopathogenic bases justifying *H. pylori* eradication in patients with functional dyspepsia are debatable, epidemiological and mainly interventional studies support this therapeutic approach. This is probably cost-effective, mainly in patients with pain-predominant dyspepsia.

References

1 Nyren O: Secretory abnormalities in functional dyspepsia. Scand J Gastroenterol 1991; 182(suppl):25–28.
2 Collen MJ, Loebenberg MJ: Basal gastric acid secretion in nonulcer dyspepsia with or without duodenitis. Dig Dis Sci 1989;34:246–250.
3 Nyren O, Adami HO, Gustavsson S, Lindgren PG, Loof L, Nyberg A: The 'epigastric distress syndrome'. A possible disease entity identified by history and endoscopy in patients with nonulcer dyspepsia. J Clin Gastroenterol 1987; 9:303–309.
4 Misra SP, Broor SL: Is gastric acid responsible for the pain in patients with essential dyspepsia? J Clin Gastroenterol 1990;12:624–627.
5 Samsom M, Verhagen MA, van Berge Henegouwen GP, Smout AJ: Abnormal clearance of exogenous acid and increased acid sensitivity of the proximal duodenum in dyspeptic patients. Gastroenterology 1999;116:515–520.
6 Bortolotti M, Brunelli F, Sarti P, Mari C, Miglioli M: Effect of omeprazole on interdigestive gastroduodenal motility of patients with ulcer-like dyspepsia. Hepatogastroenterology 1999; 46:588–593.
7 Farup PG, Hovde O, Torp R, Wetterhus S: Patients with functional dyspepsia responding to omeprazole have a characteristic gastro-oesophageal reflux pattern. Scand J Gastroenterol 1999;34:575–579.
8 Labo G, Bortolotti M, Vezzadini P, Bonora G, Bersani G: Interdigestive gastroduodenal motility and serum motilin levels in patients with idiopathic delay in gastric emptying. Gastroenterology 1986;90:20–26.
9 Malagelada JR, Stanghellini V: Manometric evaluation of functional upper gut symptoms. Gastroenterology 1985;88:1223–1231.
10 Bassoti G, Pelli MA, Morelli A: Duodenojejunal motor activity in patients with chronic dyspeptic symptoms. J Clin Gastroenterol 1990; 12:17–21.
11 Pieramico O, Ditschuneit H, Malfertheiner P: Gastrointestinal motility in patients with non-ulcer dyspepsia: A role for *Helicobacter pylori* infection? Am J Gastroenterol 1993;88:364–368.
12 Camilleri M, Malagelada JR, Kao PC, Zinsmeister AR: Gastric and autonomic responses to stress in functional dyspepsia. Dig Dis Sci 1986;31:1169–1177.
13 Von Arnim U, Domínguez-Muñoz JE, Linke A, Malfertheiner P: Association between *Helicobacter pylori* infection and bacterial overgrowth of the small intestine in non-ulcer dyspepsia. Gastroenterology 1996;110:A287.

14 Jian R, Ducrot F, Ruskone A, Chaussade S, Rambaud JC, Modigliani R, et al: Symptomatic, radionuclide and therapeutic assessment of chronic idiopathic dyspepsia. A double-blind, placebo-controlled evaluation of cisapride. Dig Dis Sci 1989;34:657–664.
15 Troncon LEA, Bennet RJM, Ahluwalia NK, Thompson DG: Abnormal intragastric distribution of food during gastric emptying in functional dyspepsia patients. Gut 1994;35:327–332.
16 Jebbink RJ, van Berge-Henegouwen GP, Akkermans LM, Amout AJ: Antroduodenal manometry: 24-hour ambulatory monitoring versus short-term stationary manometry in patients with functional dyspepsia. Eur J Gastroenterol Hepatol 1995;7:109–116.
17 Corinaldesi R, Stanghellini V, Raiti C, Rea E, Salgemini R, Barbara L: Effect of chronic administration of cisapride on gastric emptying of a solid meal and on dyspeptic symptoms in patients with idiopathic gastroparesis. Gut 1990;28:300–305.
18 Talley NJ, Shuter B, McCrudden G, Jones M, Hoschi R, Piper DW: Lack of association between gastric emptying of solid and symptoms in nonulcer dyspepsia. J Clin Gastroenterol 1989;11:625–630.
19 Davis RH, Clench MH, Mathias JR: Effects on domperidone in patients with chronic unexplained upper gastrointestinal symptoms. A double-blind, placebo-controlled study. Dig Dis Sci 1988;33:1505–1511.
20 Tack J, Broeckaert D, Coulie B, Janssens J: The influence of cisapride on gastric tone and the perception of gastric distension. Aliment Pharmacol Ther 1998;12:761–766.
21 Manes G, Domínguez-Muñoz JE, Leodolter A, Martínez S, Malfertheiner P: Does cisapride influence gastric sensitivity, compliance and duodenogastric reflexes? (abstract). Gastroenterology 1997;112:A781.
22 Mearin F, Cucala M, Azpiroz F, Malagelada JR: The origin of symptoms on the brain-gut axis in functional dyspepsia. Gastroenterology 1991;101:999–1006.
23 Bradette M, Pare P, Douville P, Morin A: Visceral perception in health and functional dyspepsia. Crossover study of gastric distension with placebo and domperidone. Dig Dis Sci 1991;36:52–58.
24 Leman M, Dederding JP, Flourie B, Franchisseur C, Rambaud JC, Jian R: Abnormal perception of visceral pain in response to gastric distension in chronic idiopathic dyspepsia. The irritable stomach syndrome. Dig Dis Sci 1991;36:1249–1254.
25 Holtmann G, Talley NJ, Goebell H: Association between *Helicobacter pylori*, duodenal mechanosensory thresholds, and small intestinal motility in chronic unexplained dyspepsia. Dig Dis Sci 1996;41:1285–1291.
26 Trimble KC, Farouk R, Pryyde A, Douglas S, Heading RC: Heightened visceral sensation in functional gastrointestinal disease is not site-specific. Evidence for a generalised disorder of gut sensitivity. Dig Dis Sci 1995;40:1607–1613.
27 Holtmann G, Goebell H, Talley NJ: Functional dyspepsia and irritable bowel syndrome: Is there a common pathophysiological basis? Am J Gastroenterol 1997;92:954–959.
28 Mertz H, Fullerton S, Naliboff B, Mayer EA: Symptoms and visceral perception in severe functional and organic dyspepsia. Gut 1998;42:814–822.
29 Klatt S, Pieramico O, Guethner C, Glasbrenner B, Beckh K, Adler G: Gastric hypersensitivity in nonulcer dyspepsia: An inconsistent finding. Dig Dis Sci 1997;42:720–723.
30 Feinle C, Meier O, Otto B, D'Amato M, Fried M: Role of duodenal lipid and cholecystokinin A receptors in the pathophysiology of functional dyspepsia. Gut 2001;48:347–355.
31 Barbera R, Feinle C, Read NW: Abnormal sensitivity to duodenal lipid infusion in patients with functional dyspepsia. Eur J Gastroenterol Hepatol 1995;11:1051–1057.
32 Greenbaum DS, Mayle JE, Vanegeren LE, Jerome JA, Mayor JW, Greenbaum RB, et al: Effects of desipramine on irritable bowel syndrome compared with atropine and placebo. Dig Dis Sci 1987;32:257–266.
33 Delvaux M, Louvel D, Mamet JP, Campos-Oriola R, Frexinos J: The kappa agonist fedotozine relieves hypersensitivity to colonic distension in patients with irritable bowel syndrome. Gastroenterology 1999;116:38–45.
34 Roman FJ, Lanet S, Hamon J, Brunelle G, Maurin A, Champeroux P, et al: Pharmacological properties of trimebutine and N-monodesmethyltrimebutine. J Pharmacol Exp Ther 1999;289:1391–1397.
35 Gershon MD: Roles played by 5-hydroxytryptamine in the physiology of the bowel. Aliment Pharmacol Ther 1999;13(suppl 2):15–30.
36 Coehlo AM, Fioramonti J, Bueno L: Mast cell degranulation induces delayed rectal allodynia in rats: Role of histamine and 5-HT. Dig Dis Sci 1998;43:727–737.
37 Tack J, Piessevaux H, Coulie B, Caenepeel P, Janssens J: Role of impaired gastric accommodation to a meal in functional dyspepsia. Gastroenterology 1998;115:1346–1352.
38 Camilleri M, Northcutt AR, Kong S, et al: Efficacy and safety of alosetron on responses to colonic distension in patients with irritable bowel syndrome. A randomised placebo-controlled trial. Lancet 2000;355:1035–1040.
39 Prather CM, Camilleri M, Zinsmeister AR, McKinzie S, Thomforde G: Tegaserod accelerates orocecal transit in patients with constipation-predominant irritable bowel syndrome. Gastroenterology 2000;118:463–468.
40 Parente F, Maconi G, Sangaletti O, Minguzzi M, Vago L, Bianchi-Porro G: Behaviour of acid secretion, gastrin release, serum pepsinogen I and gastric emptying of liquids over six months from eradication of *Helicobacter pylori* in duodenal ulcer patients. A controlled study. Gut 1995;37:210–215.
41 Sumii M, Sumii K, Tari A, Kawaguchi K, Yamamoto G, Fukino Y, et al: Expression of antral gastrin and somatostatin mRNA in *Helicobacter pylori* infected subjects. Am J Gastroenterol 1994;89:1515–1519.
42 Moss SF, Calam J: Acid secretion and sensitivity to gastrin in patients with duodenal ulcer: Effect of eradication of *Helicobacter pylori*. Gut 1993;34:888–892.
43 Hamlet A, Olbe L: The influence of *Helicobacter pylori* infection on postprandial duodenal acid load and duodenal bulb pH in humans. Gastroenterology 1996;111:391–400.
44 Pieramico O, Ditschuneit H, Malfertheiner P: Gastrointestinal motility in patients with nonulcer dyspepsia: A role for *Helicobacter pylori* infection. Am J Gastroenterol 1993;88:364–368.
45 Mearin F, de Ribot X, Balboa A, Salas A, Varas MJ, Cucala M, et al: Does Helicobacter infection increase gastric sensitivity in functional dyspepsia? Gut 1995;37:47–51.
46 Domínguez-Muñoz JE, Malfertheiner P: Effect of *Helicobacter pylori* infection on gastrointestinal motility, pancreatic secretion and hormone release in asymptomatic humans. Scand J Gastroenterol 2001, in press.
47 Armstromg D: *Helicobacter pylori* infection and dyspepsia. Scand J Gastroenterol 1996;215(suppl):38–47.
48 Moayyedi P, Soo S, Deeks J, Delaney B, Harris A, Innes M, et al: Eradication of *Helicobacter pylori* for non-ulcer dyspepsia (Cochrane review); in: The Cochrane Library, Issue 3, Oxford, Update Software, 2000.
49 Malfertheiner P, Fischbach W, Layer P, Moessner J, Stolte M, Leodolter A, et al: ELAN study proves symptomatic benefit of *Helicobacter pylori* eradication in functional dyspepsia. Gastroenterology 2000;118:A440.

Review Article

Digestive Diseases

Dig Dis 2001;19:201–211

Role of Stress in Functional Gastrointestinal Disorders

Evidence for Stress-Induced Alterations in Gastrointestinal Motility and Sensitivity

H. Mönnikes[a] J.J. Tebbe[b] M. Hildebrandt[a] P. Arck[a] E. Osmanoglou[a] M. Rose[a] B. Klapp[a] B. Wiedenmann[a] I. Heymann-Mönnikes[a]

[a]Department of Medicine, Charité, Campus Virchow-Klinikum, Humboldt-Universität zu Berlin, and
[b]Department of Internal Medicine, Philipps-Universität, Marburg, Germany

Key Words

Stress · Functional gastrointestinal disorder · Visceral sensitivity · Gastrointestinal motility · Irritable bowel syndrome

Abstract

Psychological stress is widely believed to play a major role in functional gastrointestinal (GI) disorders, especially irritable bowel syndrome (IBS), by precipitating exacerbation of symptoms. The available data clearly demonstrate that inhibition of gastric emptying and stimulation of colonic transit is the most consistent pattern in the motility response of the GI tract to acute or short-term stress. Thus, one might propose that these alterations might play a pathophysiological role in dyspeptic symptoms and alterations in stool frequency and consistency in patients with stress-related functional GI disorders. Taken together, the above-mentioned studies suggest that the colonic motor response to stress is exaggerated in IBS. There is evidence that an increased emotional response is associated with this difference in colonic, and perhaps also gastric motor responses to certain stressors. However, almost no valid data are available so far from human studies addressing the question if differences in motility responses to stress between patients with functional GI disorders and healthy subjects are due to an altered stress response associated with an imbalance of the autonomic nervous system or increased stress susceptibility. We can summarize that in experimental animals the most consistent pattern of GI motor alterations induced by various psychological and physical stressors is that of delaying gastric emptying and accelerating colonic transit. Endogenous corticotropin-releasing factor (CRF) in the brain plays a significant role in the central nervous system mediation of stress-induced inhibition of upper GI and stimulation of lower GI motor function through activation of brain CRF receptors. The inhibition of gastric emptying by CRF may be mediated by interaction with the CRF-2 receptor, while CRF-1 receptors are involved in the colonic and anxiogenic responses to stress. Endogenous serotonin, peripherally released in response to stress, seems to be involved in stress- and central CRF-induced stimulation of colonic motility by acting on 5HT-3 receptors. Taken together, the limited data available from investigations in healthy subjects and patients with functional GI disorders provide some evidence that stress affects visceral sensitivity in humans. Acute psychological stress seems to facilitate increased sensitivity to experimental visceral

KARGER

Fax +41 61 306 12 34
E-Mail karger@karger.ch
www.karger.com

0257–2753/01/0193–0201$17.50/0

Accessible online at:
www.karger.com/journals/ddi

Hubert Mönnikes, MD
Department of Medicine, Divisions of Hepatology and Gastroenterology/Psychosomatic Medicine and Psychotherapy, Universitätsklinikum Charité, Campus Virchow-Klinikum
Humboldt-Universität zu Berlin, Augustenburger Platz 1, D–13353 Berlin (Germany)
Tel. +49 30 450 553 391, Fax +49 30 450 553 991, E-Mail hubert.moennikes@charite.de

stimuli, if the stressor induces a significant emotional change. In summary, studies in experimental animals suggest that stress-induced visceral hypersensitivity is centrally mediated by endogenous CRF and involvement of structures of the emotional motor system, e.g. the amygdala. Stress-induced activation or sensitization of mucosal mast cells in the GI tract seem to be involved in stress-associated alterations of visceral sensitivity.

Introduction

The association of emotional problems with disturbances in gastrointestinal (GI) function that cause discomfort has been part of 'conventional wisdom' for many centuries [for a historical review see, 1]. Anecdotal clinical observations by Beaumont and Beaumont [2] and Cabanis et al. [3] that sadness, fear and anger affect gastric function in man, suggesting that the brain modulates the physiologic function of the GI tract, have intrigued researchers for several decades. The pioneer experimental work of Pavlov [4] and Cannon [5] in experimental animals clearly demonstrated brain–gut interactions, and the response of the GI tract to stress is perhaps the most extensively studied phenomenon of the brain–gut axis.

Stress, defined as an acute threat to the homeostasis of an organism by real (physical, 'interoceptive'; e.g. hemorrhage, gut infection) or perceived (psychological, 'exteroceptive') events, initiates adaptive physiologic and behavioral responses that serve to defend the stability of the internal environment [6–8]. Allostasis, i.e. the ability to actively maintain homeostasis through the activation of neural, endocrine and immune response systems, ensures survival of the organism. However, activation of the allostatic systems can become maladaptive due to frequent, chronic or excessive stress, which is referred to as 'allostatic load' and predisposes the acquirement of new diseases or the exacerbation of an existing disease process [9, 10].

Functional GI disorders represent a combination of chronic or recurrent GI symptoms and cannot be explained by structural or biochemical abnormalities. The link between functional GI disorders and psychosocial factors, particularly psychological, is evident based on (i) physiological studies demonstrating changes in GI function related to stress; (ii) a temporal relationship between life events and GI symptoms; (iii) epidemiological studies, and (iv) the response of patients with functional GI disorders to psychological interventions or drugs which influence emotional well being [11]. However, psychological or exteroceptive stressors differ in respect to their role as (i) a risk factor to develop a functional GI disorder later in life (early life stress like neglect, increasing disease vulnerability due to permanent enhancement of stress responsiveness); (ii) a trigger factor for onset or exacerbation of symptoms throughout life (psychosocial stressors like threatening life events, inducing transient changes in stress responsiveness), or (iii) a perpetuating factor causing symptom chronicity in patients with a functional GI disorder by triggering stress responses in initially not stressful situations (conditioned stressors, e.g. fear responses to symptoms related to a functional disease) [for review see, 12].

Central Circuitry of Stress Response

In recent years an understanding of the mechanisms underlying brain–gut interactions, particularly under conditions of acute and chronic stress, has evolved, and has enabled considerable progress in the understanding of the biological mechanisms by which psychological factors, like exteroceptive stress, translate into physiological responses relevant for GI function and how allostatic load might cause disturbed gut function or gut symptoms.

It has been proposed that an integrative network of brain structures, involving hypothalamic subnuclei (in particular the paraventricular nucleus), the periaqueductal grey, the locus coeruleus and the amygdala mediate the stress response by providing output to pontomedullary areas and to the pituitary, which in turn modulate efferent autonomic and neuroendocrine control mechanisms of the organisms. This central network receives input from cortical structures, like the medial prefrontal and the anterior cingulate cortex, as well as information from the periphery by ascending projections from the brain stem, which relay information transmitted to the brain via afferent neuronal projections and circulating substances, like glucocorticoids. Major outputs of this brain circuitry (named the 'emotional motor system' and activated in response to various stressors) to the periphery involve autonomic (autonomic nervous system), neuroendocrine (hypothalamic-pituitary-adrenal axis), and pain modulatory systems [for detailed review see, 12].

Table 1. Effects of stress on various parameters of GI motility in healthy controls

	Stressor	Parameter	Effects	References
Esophagus	Loud noises	Contraction amplitude	↑	Stacher et al. [15]
	Psychological, environmental	Contraction amplitude	↑	Young et al. [16]
Stomach	Vertigo (labyrinth stimulation)	Postprandial emptying	↓	Thompson et al. [17]
	Cold pain	Postprandial emptying	↓	Thompson et al. [18]
	Vertigo (labyrinth stimulation)	Postprandial antral phasic response	↓	Stanghellini et al. [19]
	Cold pain	Postprandial antral phasic response	↓	Stanghellini et al. [19]
	Psychological	Postprandial emptying	→	Cann et al. [20]
Small intestine	Sustained mental	Fasting MMC (frequency)	↓	McRae et al. [21]
	Psychological	Transit	↑	Cann et al. [20]
	Video game, intense driving	Fasting MMC (frequency)	↓	Valori et al. [22]
	Psychological	Transit time	↓	Ditto et al. [23]
Colon	Psychological	Contractile activity	↑	Almy et al. [24]
	Various (ice water, strobe test, ball sorting)	Spike potentials	↑	Narducci et al. [25]
	Various (ice water, strobe test, ball sorting)	Contractile activity	↑	Narducci et al. [25]

MMC = Migrating motor complex. ↑ = Increase, ↓ = decrease, → = no change.

Altered GI Motility and Sensitivity in Functional GI Disorders

A large body of evidence, mainly from studies in experimental animals, suggests that the central nervous system (CNS) response to stress modulates the autonomic nervous system outflow, activates the hypothalamic-pituitary-adrenal axis and alters pain modulatory mechanisms; these effects can be associated with changes in GI motility and visceral sensitivity. Among the various functional GI disorders, the role of stress in the pathogenesis and clinical presentation of symptoms has been most extensively studied in the irritable bowel syndrome (IBS). Thus, this article reviews evidence for the involvement of stress-induced alterations in GI motility and visceral sensitivity in the genesis of symptoms in IBS patients. In addition, the article focuses on neurobiological mechanisms mediating stress-induced changes in GI motility and visceral sensitivity, which are mainly derived from work in experimental animal models.

Effects of Stress on GI Motility in Healthy Controls

There is a considerable amount of data showing that symptoms of IBS are at least partially related to abnormal GI motility [13, 14]. While acute stress can be studied conveniently, the effects of chronic stress on the GI tract are more difficult to analyze. Thus, in the vast majority of studies on the effects of stress on GI motility in healthy controls, and also in patients, acute stressors were employed. These studies found that stress induces differential motor effects on the upper and lower GI tract in healthy human subjects. Acute psychological and physical stressors have been shown to increase contractile activity of the esophagus [15, 16]. In most studies, stress paradigms, like cold pain, labyrinth stimulation, or psychological stress result in an inhibition of gastric emptying and the postprandial antral phasic motor response [17–20], as well as a reduction in the incidence and frequency of fasting migrating motor complexes [21, 22]. However, other studies reported a stimulation of intestinal transit in response to psychological stress [20, 23]. Also, it is well established that acute physical stress (e.g. hand immersion in cold water) and psychological stress (e.g. dichotomous listening,mental arithmetic) stimulate propulsive colonic motor function in healthy subjects [24–27] (table 1, 2).

One experimental study determined whether the quality of the stimulus has an impact on the colonic motor response to stress. Psychological stress was induced by a dichotomous listening test and physical stress by hand immersion in cold water. Psychological stress induced more propagated contractions, whereas physical stress induced more simultaneous contractions suggesting that

Table 2. Effects of stress on various parameters of GI motility in healthy controls and IBS patients

	Stressor	Parameter	Effects		References
			healthy controls	IBS	
Esophagus	Mental	Contraction amplitude	↑	↑	Ayres et al. [32]
	Mental	Contraction frequency	↓	↓	Soffer et al. [33]
Stomach	Anger stressor	Antral motor activity	↑	↓	Welgan et al. [37]
Small intestine	Various mental stressors	MMC	↓	↓	Kumar and Wingate [34]
		One or more motor abnormalities	–	+	
	Two mental stressors	Duodenal phase-2 of the MMC	↓	↓	Kellow et al. [35]
		Jejunal phase-2 of the MMC	↓	(↓)	
Colon	Various (ice water, strobe test, ball sorting)	Spike potentials	↑	↑	Narducci et al. [25]
		Contractile activity	↓	↑	
	Fear, cold pressure	Motor activity	↑	↑	Welgan et al. [26]
	Mental arithmetic	2–4 cpm slow wave activity	↓	↑	
	Anger stressors	Motor activity	↑	↑↑	Welgan et al. [27]
		Spike activity	↑	↑↑	
	Mental	Motility index	→	↑	Fukudo et al. [31]

MMC = Migrating motor complex. ↑ = Increase, ↓ = decrease, (↓) = nonsignificant decrease, → = no change; + = yes, – = no.

GI motor responses to stress may vary depending on the nature of the stressor. However, in other studies these differential effects of various physical and psychological stressors on the electrical or contractile activity of the colon in healthy controls or IBS patients were not observed [26].

Taken together, the available data clearly demonstrate that inhibition of gastric emptying and stimulation of colonic transit is the most consistent pattern in the motility response of the GI tract to acute or short-term stress. Thus, one might propose that these alterations might play a pathophysiological role in dyspeptic symptoms and alterations in stool frequency and consistency in patients with stress-related functional GI disorders. This idea is supported by indirect evidence from long-term studies in healthy volunteers which showed that chronic stress causes symptoms consistent with the diagnosis of a functional GI disorder [28]. Nevertheless, the effects of chronic stress on GI motility in otherwise healthy subjects still need to be investigated further. However, this approach to reach a better understanding of the pathophysiological mechanisms underlying symptoms in functional GI disorders has not only technical but also ethical limitations. Studies in appropriate experimental animal models might be a way to approach these questions.

Effects of Stress on GI Motility in IBS

The role of stress and stressful events is well recognized in patients with functional GI disorders. Psychological stress is widely believed to play a major role in IBS by precipitating exacerbation of symptoms. Stress scores are significantly correlated with the number of disability days and of clinical visits for bowel symptoms [11, 29, 30]. As outlined above, studies investigating the effects of stress in healthy subjects and experimental animals clearly demonstrate that various types of psychological and physical stress induce alterations in GI motility, which in turn could cause abdominal symptoms and altered stool habits.

This raises the question whether GI motility responses to stress differ between healthy controls, normally free of GI symptoms, and patients with a functional GI disorder, suffering from chronic or recurrent abdominal complaints. The majority of studies addressing this question have been performed in patients with IBS and suggest differences in the gastric and colonic but not the esophageal and intestinal motor responses to stress between healthy subjects and patients (table 2).

The available body of literature nearly unanimously reports an increased colonic motor response to various psychological (e.g. strobe test, fear, mental arithmetic) and physical (e.g. ice water and cold pressure tests) stressors, as determined by different parameters of colonic motor activity (e.g. spike and 2–4 cpm slow-wave activity, contractile and motor activity) in IBS patients in comparison to healthy controls [25–27, 31]. In contrast, under stress conditions no convincing differences in esophageal and intestinal motility have been described between these two groups [32–35].

The effectiveness of an experimental stressor to produce a significantly more pronounced motor response to stress in IBS patients in comparison to controls seems to be dependent on the ability of the stressor to induce a strong emotional response, like anger [27]. In this context, it is worthwhile to mention that in 1934 Hall [36] established the use of a defecation score as an index of emotionality in rats exposed to unfamiliar surroundings. Further, it has been reported that stress induces a significantly higher colonic motor response in IBS than in controls, which was correlated with EEG power spectral changes, suggesting that the patients might have an exaggerated responsiveness to stress [31].

In IBS patients anger stress also inhibits antral motility, which was not observed in controls. This observation could be due to the fact that the anger stressor induced a more pronounced emotional response in patients than in healthy subjects [37], since several other studies clearly demonstrated an inhibition of gastric motor activity and postprandial emptying in healthy controls in response to various physical stressors [17–19]. Yet, the groups did not differ in their response to the standardized anger stressor. Thus, it cannot be ruled out that the difference in the antral motor response between the two groups is specific in IBS patients [37]. In addition, studies in patients with functional dyspepsia (FD) also showed an inhibition of propulsive gastric motor activity in response to stress [38]. Thus, one could speculate that a stress-related reduction in gastric motility might be one of the principle pathophysiological mechanisms involved in the genesis of dyspeptic symptoms in various functional GI disorders.

Taken together, the above-mentioned studies suggest that the colonic motor response to stress is exaggerated in IBS. The mechanisms underlying this difference in comparison to healthy subjects are so far not well understood, and data addressing this point are scarce. There is evidence that an increased emotional response is associated with this difference in colonic, and perhaps also gastric motor responses to certain stressors. This idea is in agreement with results of EEG studies suggestive of an exaggerated responsiveness of the brain and the colon to stress in IBS. In contrast, the available data do not support the idea that the stress-induced modulations of esophageal or intestinal motility are different between IBS patients and controls. Thus, one might speculate that the genesis of stress-related symptoms in functional GI disorders, like IBS, are at least partially due to differential motility responses throughout the various regions of the GI tract. It has been proposed that persistent alterations in autonomic responsiveness play a role in altered gastric emptying and colonic transit in the most common functional GI disorders, IBS and FD, but also in many of the extraintestinal complaints reported by such patients [12, 39]. However, almost no valid data are available so far from human studies addressing the question whether differences in motility responses to stress between patients with functional GI disorders and healthy subjects are due to an altered stress response associated with an imbalance of the autonomic nervous system or increased stress susceptibility.

Mechanisms of Stress Effects on GI Motility in Experimental Animals

The observations of these studies in healthy volunteers and patients with functional GI disorders are in good agreement with studies in experimental animals showing that delayed gastric emptying is commonly induced by various acute stressors (e.g. operant avoidance, water avoidance, acoustic stimulation, and also physical stressors like hemorrhage, abdominal surgery) in different experimental animals (among others in mice, rats, dogs, and monkeys) [40–42]. In contrast to data from the few studies available investigating this parameter in humans [28], stress inhibits intestinal transit in most experimental stress models (e.g. ether, cold water swim, restraint stress) in rats [43]. In accordance with the above-mentioned observations in humans, colonic transit, colonic motility and defecation are stimulated by the various stressors investigated so far (e.g. conditioned fear paradigm, water avoidance stress, restraint or open field stress) [40–42]. After specific stimuli, differential patterns of motility responses are also encountered; e.g. acute exposure to cold activates both gastric and colonic transit in rats [42]. However, the most consistent pattern of GI motor alterations resulting from acute exposure to physical and psychological stress, and also from activation of the immune system, is that of delayed gastric emptying and accelerated colonic transit [40, 42].

Considering the fact that IBS predominantly affects women and that symptoms consistent with IBS are most prevalent in patients with functional GI disorders, it is interesting to note that female rats are more sensitive to the effects of stress on intestinal transit than male rats, and that the colon seems to be more responsive to the effects of stress on motor activity than the upper GI tract [44–46].

The close parallelism between the effects of acute stress on GI motility in humans and experimental animals suggests that the central and peripheral pathways mediating the stress effects on GI motility delineated so far in experimental animals are similar in humans. It is well established that corticotropin-releasing factor (CRF) is one of the principle mediators in the central stress response of the organism. Among other brain areas, CRF neurons are located in the paraventricular nucleus of the hypothalamus, the amygdala and the locus coeruleus complex, which are part of the emotional motor system [12, 40, 41, 47]. Several convergent findings suggest that the stress-induced inhibition of gastric emptying and stimulation of propulsive colonic motor function is mediated by activation of brain CRF receptors in brain nuclei which are part of the emotional motor system [41, 42, 48–50]. Peripheral autonomic pathways convey acute stress and central CRF-induced inhibition of gastric emptying and stimulation of colonic motor function, whereas associated activation of the pituitary-adrenal axis does not play a role [40].

Recent studies showed that medullary CRF-2 receptors play a role in the inhibition of gastric emptying. In contrast, the experimental data point to a role of cerebral CRF-1 receptors in the stimulation of colonic transit by psychological stress or centrally injected CRF [51, 52]. Several studies in healthy subjects and IBS patients suggest that emotions like anxiety or anger are associated with GI symptoms and alterations in GI motility in response to stress [26–28, 37]. Thus, novel findings suggesting that anxiogenic behavioral responses to stress or central administration of CRF are also mediated by cerebral CRF-1 receptors [53] could be of significant relevance for the understanding of the brain pathways involved in the CNS mediation of stress-related symptoms in functional GI disorders, especially in patients with primarily or reactively associated psychological symptoms. Therefore, a recent report that treatment with a CRF-1 receptor antagonist has beneficial effects on depressive symptoms [54], might also be of relevance for the development of future treatment strategies in patients with functional GI disorders who have manifest psychological alterations, like anxiety or depression, associated with symptoms of altered bowel motor function [42, 55].

On the other hand, treatment of stress-related symptoms in functional GI disorders by targeting the peripheral pathways involved in the mediation of altered GI function under such conditions might be of advantage to avoid unwanted CNS effects. There is considerable evidence suggesting that peripheral release of serotonin (5-HT) is involved in stress- and central CRF-mediated alterations in GI function causing symptoms in patients with functional GI disorders [55–57]. Studies in experimental animals recently showed that CRF released from the CNS by stress peripherally promotes the release of 5-HT which stimulates propulsive bowel function through the 5-HT3 receptor [58, 59]. Thus, treatment of symptoms due to exaggerated bowel motility related to stress or an enhanced stress response in patients with functional GI disorders, especially IBS, are most likely a good indication for pharmacological treatments targeting 5-HT3 receptors in the GI tract [60].

Future studies in experimental animals investigating the effects of chronic stress on GI motor function might provide additional insight into the molecular mechanisms involved in the role of stress in the pathogenesis of functional GI disorders, like FD and IBS [61]. Also studies in models allowing the determination of the influence of early postnatal stressful life events, which have been shown to alter the central CRF responsiveness to stress in adulthood, could provide some insight into the neurobiological basis of the likelihood of developing a functional GI disorder [30, 45, 91].

We can summarize that in experimental animals the most consistent pattern of GI motor alterations induced by various psychological and physical stressors is that of delaying gastric emptying and accelerating colonic transit. Endogenous CRF in the brain plays a significant role in the CNS mediation of stress-induced inhibition of upper GI and stimulation of lower GI motor function through activation of brain CRF receptors. The inhibition of gastric emptying by CRF may be mediated by interaction with the CRF-2 receptor, while CRF-1 receptors are involved in the colonic and anxiogenic responses to stress. The available data suggest that hypersecretion of cerebral CRF could be involved in the pathophysiology of the stress-related exacerbation of symptoms in IBS and other functional GI disorders. Thus, in the future CRF-1 antagonists might be of therapeutic value in IBS, particularly in patients with anxiety, depression and chronic stress. Endogenous 5-HT, peripherally released in response to stress, seems to be involved in stress- and central CRF-induced stimulation of colonic motility by acting on 5HT-3 receptors. Thus, 5HT-3 receptor antagonists are of considerable interest for the treatment of stress-induced GI symptoms, among other pathophysiological mechanisms resulting from stimulation of propulsive colonic motor function.

Alterations in Visceral Perception in Functional GI Disorders

Published experimental evidence from studies assessing visceral sensitivity suggests that symptoms in functional GI disorders are related to enhanced perception of visceral stimuli [13, 14]. Several groups of investigators have reported that (i) pain and discomfort thresholds for balloon distension of the esophagus, small intestine, colon, and rectosigmoid are lowered in functional GI disorders, like noncardiac chest pain, FD, and IBS [62–72]; (ii) heightened visceral sensation in functional GI disorders is not site-specific but observable in the upper and lower GI tract [66, 73], as shown for IBS patients; (iii) changes in visceral sensitivity and symptoms over time are significantly correlated [65]; (iv) a heightened perception of normal intestinal events [74], but (v) no generalized hypersensitivity to somatic stimulation occurs [67, 75]. It has been proposed that so far at least two types of 'perceptual alterations' can be distinguished in patients with functional GI disorders: (i) hypervigilance, which is an important component of the CNS response to (exteroceptive) stress, and (ii) hyperalgesia, which in patients with functional GI disorders, like IBS, could result from a lack of activation of the descending pain modulation systems, which are known to be involved in antinociceptive effects of stress for somatic stimuli [for review see, 57, 76, 77].

However, and besides these intriguing concepts, so far information about the following points derived from appropriately designed experimental studies is scarce: (i) which effects of stress on visceral sensitivity have been proven in humans; (ii) does stress have different effects on visceral sensitivity in patients with functional GI disorders, e.g. IBS and healthy subjects, and (iii) which mechanisms are involved in stress-induced alterations in visceral sensitivity.

Effects of Stress on GI Sensitivity in Healthy Controls

There is evidence from experimental studies in humans that psychological and physical stress differentially affects visceral sensation. Erckenbrecht et al. [78, 79] showed in healthy volunteers that mental stress induces visceral hypersensitivity, as determined by a significant decrease in the threshold of 'urge to defecate' during stress. This effect was long lasting, since it was still found 1 h after stress. In contrast, physical stress induced visceral hyposensitivity, since it significantly elevated the threshold during the stress period, but not thereafter. These data underline that psychological and physical stressors may differentially affect visceral sensitivity during and after the stress period. One may conclude from these data that stimulation of the CNS by psychological stress sensitizes the perception of a painful peripheral visceral stimulus, which is in accordance with the idea of hypervigilance, while hyperstimulation of peripheral somatic perception by a physical stressor triggers distraction mechanisms that lead to decreased perception, which could be mediated by an activation of antinociceptive pain-modulating mechanisms [78, 79].

However, other studies obtained contradictory results. In an experimental study in healthy volunteers, Metevier et al. [80] and Delveaux [81] did not observe visceral hypersensitivity during or after stress, either when physical cold pressure stress or when the mental stress test 'dichotomous listening' were applied. In contrast, they report an increase in the thresholds for urge to defecate and pain, which was interpreted as a result of distraction by the stimulation [80, 81]. Further, a short-term mental stress (drawing task) did not alter the thresholds for discomfort or pain at colorectal distension in volunteers [72]. This lack of effect of the stressor on visceral perception could be due to the short duration of the stress period (5 min) and/or insufficient emotional activation by the stressor used in this study [72]. The hypothesis of an association between changes in emotionality, e.g. anxiety as an interoceptive stressor, and elevated visceral sensitivity is indirectly supported by results of a study from Ford et al. [82]. They exposed healthy volunteers to progressive muscle relaxation (PMR) and dichotomous listening stress (DLS). Both conditions did not significantly affect arousal but DLS increased and PMR reduced the level of anxiety. During the mental stress increased intensity of sensations for gas and pain during sigmoid distension at various pressure levels was observed. In contrast, PMR reduced sensation of gas at least at the middle pressure level. From this study one might conclude that the emotional quality of a given experimental stimulus thought to be stressful might be crucial to affect visceral sensitivity [82].

Effects of Stress on GI Sensitivity in Functional GI Disorders

It seems surprising but until now only a few studies have investigated the effects of stress on visceral sensitivity in clinical populations. We found in a smaller study that short-term mental stress had no measurable effect on the thresholds for discomfort or pain at colorectal distension in healthy volunteers and IBS patients [72]. In contrast, the two groups investigated were different in respect to their basal pain perception thresholds, with IBS patients showing increased sensitivity under such condition and their response to a stimulus causing mental distraction. In comparison to the control group, IBS patients showed a blunted increase in the pain perception threshold during mental distraction, which is suggestive of a CNS-mediated perceptional abnormality in IBS patients which is independent of the effects of short-term stress. However, it has recently been shown for the first time that stress can induce esophageal hypersensitivity in patients with gastroesophageal reflux disease. In this study stress significantly increased the sensitivity score to esophageal acid perfusion in patients with erosive esophagitis as well as in nonerosive gastroesophageal reflux disease [83].

Taken together, the limited data available from investigations in healthy subjects and patients with functional GI disorders provide some evidence that stress affects visceral sensitivity in humans. Acute psychological stress seems to facilitate increased sensitivity to experimental visceral stimuli, if the stressor induces a significant emotional change. Alterations in the CNS modulation of visceral perception independent of the effects of acute stress on visceral sensitivity are also found in functional GI disorders, at least in IBS. Also proof of clinically relevant differences in the effect of stress on visceral sensitivity between healthy subjects and patients with functional GI disorders still needs to be established. Further, the psychological and biological mechanisms which might be involved in stress-associated alterations of visceral sensitivity in patients with functional GI disorders have not been sufficiently investigated until today. In this context it is worthwhile to mention that in a recent study multicomponent behavioral treatment in IBS patients significantly improved well-being without affecting visceral sensitivity [71].

Mechanisms of Stress Effects on GI Sensitivity in Experimental Animals

It is well established, predominantly by studies in experimental animals, that stress- and fear-induced somatic hyposensitivity is mediated by descending supra- and bulbospinal projections from the periaqueductal grey and the locus coeruleus, which modulate excitability of ascending sensory afferents by the release of various neurotransmitters – mainly noradrenaline, opioids, glutamine and 5-HT – at the spinal level. The activity of these stress-activated endogenous pain modulation systems is affected by input from the emotional motor system as mentioned above [for details see, 57, 76, 77]. Recent evidence suggests that the somatic hypoalgesia in response to stress can be accompanied by visceral hyperalgesia or hypersensitivity [84, 85]. In experimental animal studies, an increased frequency of abdominal wall contractions is an established pseudo-affective parameter to semiquantitatively determine visceral pain. In an interesting study in rats Gue et al. [85] demonstrated that after restraint stress applied for 2 h before colorectal distension, the pseudo-affective response evoked by rectal distension was significantly higher in stressed animals, suggesting that stress sensitizes the animals to the distension stimulus by inducing visceral hypersensitivity. In the same model, the effect of the stressor on somatic pain tolerance, as determined by the tail-flick paradigm, was also investigated. It was observed that stressed rats showed a greater delay in the tail-flick response up to 45 min after the end of the stress, an observation which is in good agreement with the above-mentioned phenomenon of stress-induced somatic hypoalgesia. Taken together, these observations show that in this experimental animal model stress induces visceral hypersensitivity associated with a somatic hyposensitivity. In the same model, intracerebroventricular injection of a CRF-antagonist before the distension procedure dose-dependently diminished the effect of stress on the pseudo-affective response parameter. In addition, CRF administered intracerebroventricularly dose-dependently mimicked the effect of stress on the number of abdominal contractions at rectal distension, suggesting that CRF in the brain plays a physiological role in the stress-induced sensitization of experimental animals to GI visceral stimuli. Further this group showed that peripheral administration of a mast cell stabilizer suppressed the stress- and CRF-induced hypersensitivity to rectal distension. In addition, they found that the level of histamine released from the intestines of stressed rats was significantly increased in vitro, whereas the number of mucosal mast cells was unchanged compared to the control group [85,

86]. These data suggest that intestinal mast cells become more sensitive to a mast cell degranulator after stress and reinforce the hypothesis for a role of mast cells in stress-induced visceral hypersensitivity. The sensitized mast cells may be responsible for the visceral hypersensitivity in response to stress through a higher synthesis and later on release of histamine and/or other mast cell mediators [85–87]. Despite the fact that the number of mast cells in stressed rats was unchanged compared to the control group – which is contrary to studies in IBS patients who have been shown to present more mast cells than healthy controls [88] – this idea is in agreement with neuroanatomical studies and data obtained in humans showing a close proximity of mucosal mast cells with the enteric nervous system [77]. As has been shown in humans by Santos et al. [89], experimental stress induces release of histamine and other mast cell products from the intestine. In this context, one might speculate that the beneficial effects of tricyclic antidepressants in IBS might be due to their antagonistic action on H1 and H2 receptors as well as modulation of mast cell function. This hypothesis has been supported by recent in vitro findings showing that different antidepressants inhibit histamine release from peritoneal mast cells [89].

The associated emotions are decisive for a particular stimulus to be perceived as stressful or not; situations causing high levels of anxiety have been shown to be very effective as a stressor. It has been proposed that the emotional motor cortex is involved in stress-induced hypersensitivity. The central amygdaloid nucleus is a key limbic structure and as part of the emotional motor cortex involved in the expression of anxiety as well as in autonomic and visceral function in response to stress. Stereotaxic delivery of corticosterone into the central amygdaloid nucleus increases anxiety in rats. Greenwood-Van Meerveld et al. [90] showed in this experimental model that naive rats with corticosterone implants in the amygdala and increased levels of anxiety display an exaggerated response to innocuous colorectal distension. This effect is still observed after colonic sensitization by intracolonic pretreatment with a low concentration of acetic acid. These findings suggest a relationship between anxiety, which can be regarded as an internalized stressor, and visceral hypersensitivity, which seems to be at least partially mediated through stimulation of the central amygdala.

In summary, studies in experimental animals suggest that stress-induced visceral hypersensitivity is centrally mediated by endogenous CRF and involvement of structures of the emotional motor system, e.g. the amygdala. Stress-induced activation or sensitization of mucosal mast cells in the GI tract seem to be involved in stress-associated alterations in visceral sensitivity.

References

1 Wolf S: The psyche and the stomach – A historical vignette. Gastroenterology 1981;80:605–614.
2 Beaumont W, Beaumont OW (eds): Experiments and Observations on the Gastric Juice and the Physiology of Digestion. New York, Dover Press, 1833, pp 1–280.
3 Cabanis PJG: Introduction; in Mora G, Saidi MD (eds): On the Relations between the Physical and Moral Aspects of Man. Baltimore, Johns Hopkins University Press, 1981, p 650.
4 Pavlov I: The Work of the Digestive Glands (English translation by WH Thompson). London, Criffin, 1910.
5 Cannon WB: Bodily Changes in Pain, Hunger, Fear and Rage. New York, Appleton, 1929.
6 Selye H: Syndrome produced by diverse nocuous agents. Nature 1936;138:32.
7 Selye H: Stress in Health and Disease. Boston, Butterworths, 1976, vol 6: Theories, pp 928–1148.
8 Chrousos GP, Gold PW: The concepts of stress and stress system disorders: Overview of physical and behavioral homeostasis. JAMA 2001; 1992:1244–1252.
9 McEwen BS, Seeman T: Elaborating and testing the concepts of allostasis and allostatic load. Ann NY Acad Sci 1999;896:30–47.
10 McEwen BS, Stellar E: Stress and the individual: Mechanisms leading to disease. Arch Intern Med 1993;153:2093–2101.
11 Kamm MA: The role of psychosocial factors in functional gut disease. Eur J Surg Suppl 1998; 583:37–40.
12 Mayer EA: The neurobiology of stress and gastrointestinal disease. Gut 2000;47:861–869.
13 Drossman DA, Whitehead WE, Camilleri M: Irritable bowel syndrome: A technical review for practice guideline development. Gastroenterology 1997;112:2118–2219.
14 Berstad A: Functional dyspepsia – A conceptual framework. Gut 2000;47(suppl 4):iv3–iv4.
15 Stacher G, Steinringer H, Blau A: Acoustically evoked esophageal contractions and defense reactions. Psychophysiology 1979;16:234–241.
16 Young LD, Richter JE, Anderson KO, et al: The effects of psychological and environmental stressors on peristaltic esophageal contractions in healthy volunteers. Psychophysiology 1987; 24:132–141.
17 Thompson DG, Richelson E, Malagelada J-R: Perturbation of gastric emptying and duodenal motility through the central nervous system. Gastroenterology 1982;83:1200–1206.
18 Thompson DG, Richelson E, Malagelada J-R: Perturbation of upper gastrointestinal function by cold stress. Gut 1983;24:277–283.
19 Stanghellini V, Malagelada J-R, Zinsmeister AR, Go WLW, Kao PC: Stress-induced gastroduodenal motor disturbances in humans: Possible humoral mechanisms. Gastroenterology 1983;85:83–91.
20 Cann PA, Read NW, Cammack J, Childs H, Holden S, Kashman R, Longmore J, Nix S, Simms N, Swallow K, et al: Psychological stress and the passage of a standard meal through the stomach and small intestine in man. Gut 1983; 24:236–240.
21 McRae S, Younger K, Thompson DG, Wingate DL: Sustained mental stress alters human jejunal motor activity. Gut 1982;23:404–409.
22 Valori RM, Kumar D, Wingate DL: Effects of different types of stress and of 'prokinetic' drugs on the control of the fasting motor complex in humans. Gastroenterology 1986;90: 1890–1900.

23 Ditto B, Miller SB, Barr RG: A one hour active coping stressor reduces small bowel transit time in healthy young adults. Psychosom Med 1998;60:7–10.
24 Almy TP, Kern F, Tulin FK: Alterations in colonic function in man under stress. II. Experimental production of sigmoid spasm in healthy persons. Gastroenterology 1949;12:425–428.
25 Narducci F, Snape WJ, Battle WM, London RL, Cohen S: Increased colonic motility during exposure to a stressful situation. Dig Dis Sci 1985;30:40–44.
26 Welgan P, Meshkinpour H, Hoehler F: The effect of stress on colon motor and electrical activity in irritable bowel syndrome. Psychosom Med 1985;47:139–149.
27 Welgan P, Meshkinpour H, Beeler M: The effect of anger on colon motor and myoelectric activity in irritable bowel syndrome. Gastroenterology 1988;94:1150–1156.
28 Erckenbrecht JF, Schafer R, Kohler G, Enck P: Dyspeptic symptoms in healthy volunteers with stress are related to stress induced increase of anxiety – Results of a prospective study with a longterm 'physiological' stress model. J Gastrointest Motil 1993;5:A189.
29 Wilhelmsen I: The role of psychosocial factors in gastrointestinal disorders. Gut 2000; 47(suppl 4):iv73–iv75.
30 Stam R, Akkermans LM, Wiegant VM: Trauma and the gut: Interactions between stressful experience and intestinal function. Gut 1997; 40:704–709.
31 Fukudo S, Nomura T, Muranaka M, Taguchi F: Brain-gut response to stress and cholinergic stimulation in irritable bowel syndrome. A preliminary study. J Clin Gastroenterol 1993;17:133–141.
32 Ayres RC, Smith CL, Naylot K: Stress and oesophageal motility in normal subjects and patients with irritable bowel syndrome. Gut 1989;30:1540–1543.
33 Soffer EE, Pope HG Jr, Wingate DL: Effect of stress on oesophageal motor function in normal subjects and in patients with the irritable bowel syndrome. Gut 1988;29:1591–1594.
34 Kumar D, Wingate DL: The irritable bowel syndrome: A paroxysmal motor disorder. Lancet 1985;ii:973–977.
35 Kellow JE, Langeluddecke PM, Eckersley GM, Jones MP, Tenant CC: Effects of acute psychologic stress on small-intestinal motility in health and the irritable bowel syndrome. Scand J Gastroenterol 1992;27:53–58.
36 Hall CS: Emotional behavior in the rat. I. Defecation and urination as a measure of individual differences in emotionality. J Comp Psychiatry 1934;18:385–403.
37 Welgan P, Meshkinpour H, Ma L: Role of anger in antral motor activity in irritable bowel syndrome. Dig Dis Sci 2000;45:248–251.
38 Camilleri M, Malagelada JR, Kao PC, et al: Gastric and autonomic responses to stress in functional dyspepsia. Dig Dis Sci 1986;31:1169–1177.
39 Tougas G: The autonomic nervous system in functional bowel disorders. Gut 2001;47(suppl 4):iv78–iv80.
40 Taché Y, Martinez V, Million M, Rivier J: Corticotropin-releasing factor and the brain-gut motor response to stress. Can J Gastroenterol 1999;13(suppl A):18A–25A.
41 Taché Y, Mönnikes H, Bonaz B, Rivier J: Role of CRF in stress-related alterations of gastric and colonic motor function. Ann NY Acad Sci 1993;697:233–243.
42 Taché Y, Martinez V, Million M, Wang L: Stress and the gastrointestinal tract. III. Stress-related alterations of gut motor function: Role of brain corticotropin-releasing factor receptors. Am J Physiol Gastrointest Liver Physiol 2001;280:G173–G177.
43 Williams CL, Burks TF: Stress, opioids, and gastrointestinal transit; in Taché Y, Morley J, Brown MR (eds): Hans Selye Symposia on Neuroendocrinology and Stress: Neuropeptides and Stress. New York, Springer, 1989, pp 175–187.
44 Enck P, Holtmann G: Stress and gastrointestinal motility in animals: A review of the literature. J Gastrointest Motil 1992;1:83–90.
45 Stam R, Croiset G, Akkermans LM, Wiegant VM: Sensitization of the colonic response to novel stress after previous stressful experience. Am J Physiol 1996;271:R1270–R1273.
46 Stam R, Croiset G, Akkermans LM, Wiegant VM: Effects of novelty and conditioned fear on small intestinal and colonic motility and behaviour in the rat. Physiol Behav 1995;58:803–809.
47 Valentino RJ, Miselis RR, Pavcovich LA: Pontine regulation of pelvic viscera: Pharmacological target for pelvis visceral dysfunction. Trends Pharmacol Sci 1999;20:253–260.
48 Mönnikes H, Schmidt BG, Raybould HE, Taché Y: CRF in the paraventricular nucleus mediates gastric and colonic motor response to restraint stress. Am J Physiol 1992;262:G137–G143.
49 Mönnikes H, Schmidt BG, Taché Y: Psychological stress-induced accelerated colonic transit in rats involves hypothalamic corticotropin-releasing factor. Gastroenterology 1993;104:716–723.
50 Mönnikes H, Schmidt BG, Tebbe J, Bauer C, Taché Y: Microinfusion of corticotropin releasing factor into the locus coeruleus/subcoeruleus nuclei stimulates colonic motor function in rats. Brain Res 1994;644:101–108.
51 Maillot C, Million M, Wei JY, Gauthier A, Taché Y: Peripheral corticotropin-releasing factor and stress-stimulated colonic motor activity involve type 1 receptors in rats. Gastroenterology 2000;119:1569–1579.
52 Martinez V, Taché Y: Role of CRF receptor 1 in central CRF-induced stimulation of colonic propulsion in rats. Brain Res 2001;893:29–35.
53 Steckler T, Holsboer F: Corticotropin-releasing hormone receptor subtypes and emotion. Biol Psychiatry 2001;46:1480–1508.
54 Zobel AW, Nickel T, Kunzel HE, Ackl N, Sonntag A, Ising M, Holsboer F: Effects of the high-affinity corticotropin-releasing hormone receptor 1 antagonists R121919 in major depression: The first 20 patients treated. J Psychiatr Res 2000;34:171–181.
55 Taché Y, Mönnikes H: CRF in the central nervous system mediates stress-induced stimulation of colonic motor function: Relevance to the pathophysiology of IBS; in Mayer EA, Raybould HE (eds): Basic and Clinical Aspects of Chronic Abdominal Pain, ed 1. Amsterdam, Elsevier Science, 1993, pp 141–151.
56 Mönnikes H, König M, Tebbe J, et al: Serotonin – A mediator of visceral nociception and pain with implications for functional gastrointestinal disorders; in Goebell H, Holtmann G, Talley NJ (eds): Functional Dyspepsia and Irritable Bowel Syndrome, ed 1. Lancaster, Kluwer Academic, 1998, pp 77–84.
57 Mönnikes H: Pharmacology of altered brain-gut interactions; in Corazziari E (ed): Neurogastroenterology. Berlin, de Gruyter, 1996, pp 85–108.
58 Miyata K, Kamato T, Nishida H, Ito H, Yuki H, Yamano M, Tsutsumi R, Katsuyama Y, Honda K: Role of serotonin$_3$ receptor in stress-induced defecation. J Pharmacol Exp Ther 1992;261:297–307.
59 Miyata K: Involvement of the 5-HT3 receptor in CRH induced defecation in rats. Am J Physiol Gastrointest Liver Physiol 1998;274:G827–G831.
60 Prior A, Read NW: Reduction of rectal sensitivity and postprandial motility by granisetron, a 5HT$_3$ receptor antagonist, in patients with irritable bowel syndrome (IBS). Aliment Pharmacol Ther 1993;7:175–180.
61 Bonaz B, Rivest S: Effect of a chronic stress on CRF neuronal activity and expression of its type 1 receptor in the rat brain. Am J Physiol Regul Integr Comp Physiol 1998;275:R1438–R1449.
62 Ritchie J: Pain from distention of the pelvic colon by inflating a balloon in the irritable bowel syndrome. Gut 1973;14:125–132.
63 Richter JE, Laurence MD, Bradley A: The irritable esophagus; in Mayer EA, Raybould HE (eds): Basic and Clinical Aspects of Chronic Abdominal Pain, ed 1. Amsterdam, Elsevier, 1993, pp 45–54.
64 Lembo T, Munakata J, Mertz H, Niazi N, Kodner A, Nikas V, Mayer EA: Evidence for the hypersensitivity of lumbar splanchnic afferents in irritable bowel syndrome. Gastroenterology 1994;107:1686–1696.
65 Mertz H, Naliboff B, Munakata J, Niazi N, Mayer EA: Altered rectal perception is a biological marker of patients with irritable bowel syndrome. Gastroenterology 1995;109:40–52.
66 Trimble KC, Farouk R, Pryde A, Douglas S, Heading RC: Heightened visceral sensation in functional gastrointestinal disease is not site-specific. Evidence for a generalized disorder of gut sensitivity. Dig Dis Sci 1995;40:1607–1613.
67 Whitehead WE, Holtkotter B, Enck P, et al: Tolerance for rectosigmoid distension in irritable bowel syndrome. Gastroenterology 1990; 98:1187–1192.
68 Prior A, Sorial E, Sun WM, Read N: Irritable bowel syndrome: Differences between patients who show rectal sensitivity and those who do not. Eur J Gastroenterol Hepatol 1993;5:343–349.

69 Mearin F, Cucula M, Azpiroz F, Malagelada JR: The origin of symptoms on the brain-gut-axis in functional dyspepsia. Gastroenterology 1991;101:999–1006.
70 Bradette M, Pare WP, Douvillle P: Visceral perception in health and functional dyspepsia. Crossover study of gastric distension with placebo and domperidone. Dig Dis Sci 1991;36: 52–58.
71 Heymann-Mönnikes I, Arnold R, Florin I, Herda C, Melfsen S, Mönnikes H: Evaluation of a multi-component behavioral treatment for the irritable bowel syndrome. Am J Gastroenterol 2000;62:981–994.
72 Mönnikes H, Heymann-Mönnikes I, Arnold R: Patients with irritable bowel syndrome (IBS) have alterations in the CNS-modulation of visceral afferent perception (abstract). Gut 1995; 37:A168.
73 Constantini M, Sturniolo GC, Zaninotto G, et al: Altered esophageal pain threshold in irritable bowel syndrome. Dig Dis Sci 1998;38:206–212.
74 Kellow JE, Eckersley GM, Jones BJ: Enhanced perception of physiological intestinal motility in the irritable bowel syndrome. Gastroenterology 1991;101:1621–1627.
75 Cook IJ, Van Eeden A, Collins SM: Patients with irritable bowel syndrome have greater pain tolerance than normal subjects. Gastroenterology 1987;93:727–733.
76 Mayer EA: Spinal and supraspinal modulation of visceral sensation. Gut 2000;47(suppl 4): iv69–iv72.
77 Bueno L, Fioramonti J, Delvaux M, Frexinos J: Mediators and pharmacology of visceral sensitivity: From basic to clinical investigations. Gastroenterology 1997;112:1714–1743.
78 Erckenbrecht JF: Noise and intestinal motor alterations; in Bueno L, Collins S, Junien JL (eds): Stress and Digestive Motility. London, Libbey Eurotext, 1989, pp 93–96.
79 Erckenbrecht JF: Central nervous system modulation of gastrointestinal functions. Z Gastroenterol 1993;31(suppl 5):6–9.
80 Metevier S, Delvaux M, Louvel D, et al: Influence of stress on sensory thresholds to rectal distension in healthy volunteers. Gastroenterology 1996;110:A717.
81 Delvaux M: Stress and visceral perception. Can J Gastroenterol 1999;13(suppl):32A–36A.
82 Ford MJ, Camilleri M, Zinsmeister AR, et al: Psychosensory modulation of colonic sensation in the human transverse and sigmoid colon. Gastroenterology 1995;109:1772–1780.
83 Fass R, Malagon I, Naliboff B, et al: Effect of psychologically induced stress on symptom perception and autonomic nervous system response of patients with erosive esophagitis. Gastroenterology 2000;118:A637.
84 Coutinho SV, Urban MO, Gebhart GF: Role of glutamate receptors and nitric oxide in the rostral ventromedial medulla in visceral hyperalgesia. Pain 1998;78:59–69.
85 Gue M, Del Rio Lacheze C, Eutamene H, et al: Stress-induced hypersensitivity to rectal distension in rats: Role of CRF and mast cells. Neurogastroenterol Motil 1997;9:271–279.
86 Eutamene H, Theodorou V, Vergnolle N, et al: Involvement of interleukin-1, prostaglandins and mast cells in rectal distension-induced colonic water secretion in rats. J Physiol (Lond) 1998;506:245–252.
87 Castagliuolo I, Wershil BK, Karalis K, et al: Colonic mucin release in response to immobilization stress is mast cell dependent. Am J Physiol Gastrointest Liver Physiol 1998;274: G1094–G1100.
88 Weston AP, Biddle WL, Bhatia PS, et al: Terminal ileal mucosal mast cells in irritable bowel syndrome. Dig Dis Sci 1993;38:1590–1595.
89 Santos J, Saperas E, Nogueiras C, et al: Release of mast cell mediators in the jejunum by cold pain stress in humans. Gastroenterology 1998; 114:640–648.
90 Greenwood-Van Meerveld B, Gibson M, Gunter W, Shephard J, Foreman R: Stereotaxic delivery of corticosterone to the amygdala modulates colonic sensitivity in rats. Brain Res 2001;893:135–142.
91 Continho SV, Sablad M, Miller JC, Zhou H, Lam A, Bayati AI, Plotsky PM, Mayer EA: Neonatal maternal separation results in stress-induced visceral hyperalgesia in adult rats: A new model for IBS. Neurogastroenterology Motility 2000;12:301–306.

Review Article

Digestive Diseases

Dig Dis 2001;19:212–218

Basic Pathophysiologic Mechanisms in Irritable Bowel Syndrome

Emeran A. Mayer Bruce D. Naliboff Lin Chang

UCLA/CURE Neuroenteric Disease Program, Department of Medicine, Physiology and Biobehavioral Sciences, UCLA School of Medicine, Los Angeles, Calif., USA

Key Words

Corticotropin-releasing factor · Emotional motor system · Visceral pain · Hypothalamic pituitary adrenal axis · Functional brain imaging · Animal models

Abstract

Converging evidence supports the concept that the irritable bowel syndrome (IBS) symptom complex results from altered regulation of gastrointestinal motility and epithelial function, as well as an altered perception of visceral events. Despite similar symptoms, there is likely heterogeneity of underlying dysfunction and pathogenesis in different subgroups of IBS patients: the syndrome may be produced by primary alterations in the central nervous system (CNS; top down model), or by primary alterations in the periphery (bottom up model), or by a combination of both. One plausible mechanism by which alterations in the CNS result in symptoms, is the enhanced responsiveness of central stress/emotion circuits. The physiological effects of psychological and physical stressors on gut function and brain-gut interactions are mediated by outputs of the emotional motor system in terms of autonomic, neuroendocrine, attentional and pain modulatory responses. IBS patients show an enhanced responsiveness of this system manifesting in altered modulation of gastrointestinal motility, secretion, immune function and in alterations in the perceptual and emotional response to visceral events.

This study was supported by NIH DK 48351 (E.A.M.), NR 04881 (B.D.N.) and AR 46122 (L.C.).

Introduction

Progress in the understanding of the pathophysiology and pathogenesis of irritable bowel syndrome (IBS) has been slow, and the development of effective clinically relevant drugs has made little progress during the past decade. A primary reason for this lack of progress has been the focus on descriptive and symptom-based studies, and the futile attempt to develop drugs without a generally agreed upon disease model. Most importantly, there has been no serious attempt to develop animal models with high face and construct validity. More recently, converging evidence from epidemiological and animal experimental studies on brain-gut interactions, and on the neurobiology of emotions supports a conceptual model of IBS which is based on the enhanced responsiveness of limbic circuits in the brain to stressors and emotional stimuli [for review see 1, 2]. In this model, symptoms can arise both in response to centrally acting stimuli (stress, emotions) as well as peripherally acting perturbations of the natural homeostasis (infection, inflammation).

KARGER

Fax + 41 61 306 12 34
E-Mail karger@karger.ch
www.karger.com

Accessible online at:
www.karger.com/journals/ddi

Emeran A. Mayer, MD
CURE Neuroenteric Disease Program, UCLA Division of Digestive Diseases
GLA VA HS, Bldg. 115/CURE, 11301 Wilshire Boulevard
Building 115, Room 223, Los Angeles, CA 90073 (USA)
Tel. +1 310 312 9276, Fax +1 310 794 2864, E-Mail emayer@ucla.edu

Emotion, Stress and the Gastrointestinal Tract

According to the traditional view, emotions are generated by a nonspecific system within the brain ('limbic system'). Furthermore, it has long been assumed that since the most relevant aspects of human emotions are the associated conscious feelings (fear, anxiety, sadness, disgust), emotions cannot be studied scientifically in animal models. However, recent neurobiological evidence supports the concept of distinct neural circuits generating emotion-specific patterns of autonomic and neuroendocrine modulation of the viscera and the body in general [3]. For example, preliminary evidence from brain-imaging studies suggests that the emotion of fear involves a circuit involving the amygdala complex, while the emotion of disgust involves the insula [4]. The emotion-specific activation of central circuits appears to be reflected in emotion-specific patterns of gastrointestinal (GI) tract modulation. While the emotion of anger is associated with enhanced contractions of the upper and lower GI tract, increased mucosal blood flow and enhanced gastric acid secretion, the emotion of fear is associated with inhibition of upper GI motility, and simultaneous stimulation of distal colonic function [for review see 5]. The translation of neuronal activity within emotion-specific circuits within the brain into distinct patterns of GI function is accomplished by the emotional motor system (EMS). This system generates parallel outputs in response to emotional activation in terms of autonomic, neuroendocrine, arousal and perceptual modulation of body functions (fig. 1). In the following, we will focus on one of the best characterized emotions, fear/anxiety, and the underlying biological mechanism, the stress response.

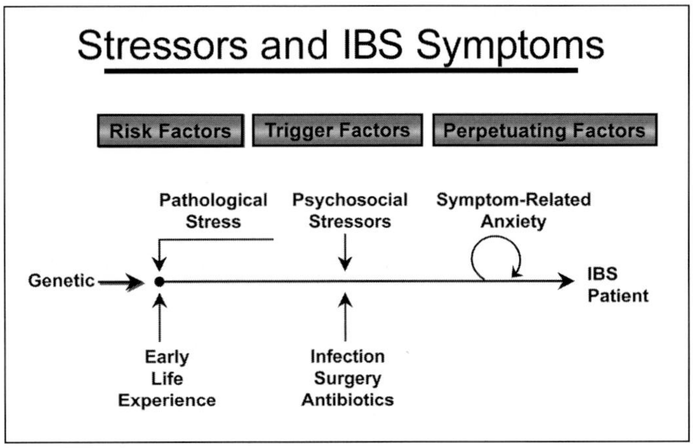

Fig. 1. Role of stress in development and modulation of IBS symptoms. Different types of stressors may play a role in the permanent biasing of stress responsiveness, in transient activation of the stress response and in the persistence of symptoms. With permission from Mayer et al. [2].

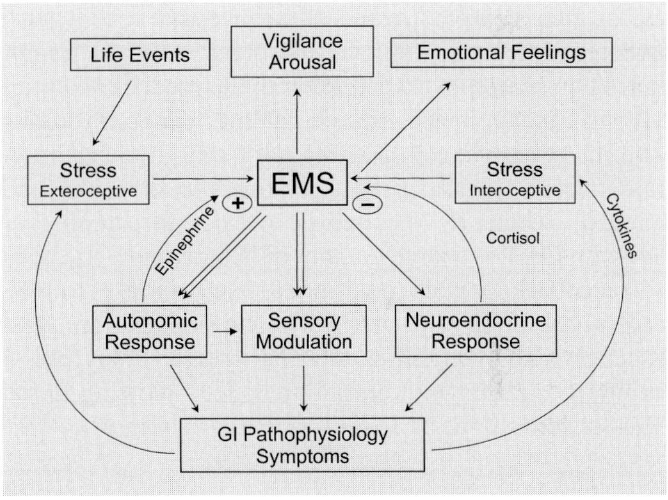

Fig. 2. Inputs and outputs of the emotional motor system (EMS). Output pathways of the EMS are activated by psychosocial (exteroceptive) and physical (interoceptive) stressors. Major outputs to the periphery are autonomic, pain modulatory and neuroendocrine responses. An important output to the forebrain occurs in terms of attentional and emotional modulation. Feedback from the gut to the EMS occurs in form of neuroendocrine (adrenaline, cortisol) as well as visceral afferent mechanisms. With permission from Mayer et al. [2].

A Variety of Stressor Types Play a Role in the Development of Irritable Bowel Syndrome

Stress, defined as an acute threat to the homeostasis of an organism, be it real (physical) or perceived (psychological), and whether posed by events in the outside world, or from within, evokes adaptive responses which serve to defend the stability of the internal environment and to assure the survival of the organism. The conscious emotional feelings associated with stress are fear, anxiety and anger. Numerous reports in the literature have provided evidence for a prominent role of stress in the pathophysiology [6] and in the clinical presentation of IBS symptoms [for review see 1, 7, 8]. The reader is referred to these articles for detailed references. A model that summarizes the possible role of different types of stressors in the development and modulation of IBS symptoms is shown in figure 2. According to this model, different types of stressors play a role in (1) permanent enhancement of stress responsiveness (pathological stress), (2) transient symptom exacerbation, and (3) symptom perpetuation (symptom-generated stress). Early life stress and trauma, in the form of abuse, neglect or loss of the primary care giver play a major role in the vulnerability of individuals to develop functional GI disorders later in life. Acute, life-threatening stress episodes in adult life (rape, post-traumatic stress disorder) are also important risk factors in the development of functional GI disorders. In the genetically predisposed individual, both early life stress and severe life-threatening stress (referred in the current review as 'pathological stressors') can result in permanent, irreversible enhancement in the responsiveness of central stress circuits and therefore vulnerability to develop functional (as well as affective) disorders later in life. Other types of stressors occurring throughout the life of an individual, which may only result in transient changes in the stress responsiveness, clearly play a role in symptom exacerbation. For example, psychosocial stressors in the form of sustained, threatening life events have been associated with the onset and symptom exacerbation in IBS. 'Physical' or interoceptive stressors of the digestive system, such as enteric infections, trauma, and surgery may play a similar role in symptom exacerbation in the predisposed individual. Finally, in the affected patient, fear conditioning and interoceptive conditioning are likely to play important roles in triggering stress responses to situations and contexts which by themselves are not threatening or stressful [9]. For a large number of IBS patients, the positive feedback loop of (conditioned) fear responses to interoceptive stimuli or contextually conditioned stimuli (associated with symptom-generating stressors) may play a primary role in symptom maintenance following initial stressor resolution.

Emotional States Are Translated into Integrative Physiological Responses of the GI Tract

The traditional concept of stress has focused on the subjective conscious feelings (fear, anxiety, anger), thoughts, beliefs and memories reported by some individuals in association with stressful life events. However, the major breakthroughs in this area have occurred through an understanding of the biological mechanisms which are responsible for the detrimental effect of certain stressful life events on health [10]. The organism's response to stress is generated by a network comprised of integrative brain structures, in particular subregions of the hypothalamus (paraventricular nucleus, PVN), amygdala and periaqueductal grey. These structures receive input from visceral and somatic afferents and from cortical structures, in particular the ventral subdivision of the anterior cingulate and the medial prefrontal (ventromedial and orbitofrontal) cortex [11, 12]. This integrative network provides outputs to the pituitary and to pontomedullary nuclei, which in turn mediate the neuroendocrine and autonomic output to the body, respectively. This central stress circuitry is under feedback control via ascending monoaminergic projections from these brainstem nuclei, in particular serotonergic (raphe nuclei) and noradrenergic (NA; including locus coeruleus) nuclei, and via circulating glucocorticoids, which exert an inhibitory control via central glucocorticoid receptors located in the medial prefrontal cortex and hippocampus [13]. The parallel outputs of this central circuitry (EMS) which is activated in response to various stressors include responses of the autonomic nervous system, the hypothalamus-pituitary-adrenal (HPA) axis, endogenous pain modulatory systems and ascending aminergic pathways. These pathways are summarized in figure 1.

One important chemical mediator of the central stress response is corticotropin-releasing factor (CRF; and probably related molecules such as urocortin and currently unknown molecules) located in certain effector neurons of the PVN, the amygdala, and the locus coeruleus complex [14]. CRF secretion by PVN neurons is under positive feedback regulation by central NA pathways (including those originating from locus coeruleus), thereby forming a bi-directional positive feedback loop between the CRF-NA systems. Central injection of CRF can reproduce behavioral and physiologic responses similar to those seen in response to acute psychological stress [15, 16]. Similarly, inhibition of CRF-mediated responses by antagonists [6, 15], or interference with the CRF system in knock out animals, results in a decrease in the animals' response to stress [17, 18].

Enhanced Responsiveness of Central Stress Circuits

The responsiveness of the EMS is likely to be under partial genetic control and shows considerable plasticity in response to early life events [19] and to certain types of pathological stress [20]. For example, studies in animals and men have clearly demonstrated that certain types of pathological stress can alter the responsiveness of feedback systems by downregulation of pre- and/or postsynaptic receptors (adrenergic, serotonergic, glucocorticoid receptors) and in the most severe forms by structural changes in certain brain regions [for review see 1]. Thus, pathological stress cannot only activate, but also fundamentally change the responsiveness and output of the central stress circuits. These alterations could affect the individual output pathways of the EMS differentially and in different directions; e.g., an increase or decrease in target-specific sympathetic and vagal outputs, up- or downregulation of the HPA axis, and up- or downregulation of pain perception. Some of the best characterized alterations in this central adaptation to pathological stress are an increase in CRF synthesis and secretion [16], an increase in the activity and sensitivity of central NA systems [19, 21], and downregulation of glucocorticoid receptors [22] suggestive of an enhanced HPA response to stress. As a consequence of these alterations in the central stress circuitry, secondary changes in receptor systems can occur in spinal or peripheral target cells of the output systems. Thus, in cases of pathological stress resulting in permanent changes in the central stress circuitry, lifelong changes in peripheral receptor systems may also be expected. In the following, we will discuss evidence for alterations in the three output systems of the EMS in IBS patients.

Changes in Autonomic Nervous System Responses

In the healthy organism, the EMS generates distinct, emotion-specific patterns of autonomic nervous system activity which are reflected in distinct emotion-specific activity patterns of the GI tract (see above). The acute modulation of motility, epithelial function (secretion) and blood flow is accomplished by (1) the different branches of the efferent vagus nerve (modulating gastric, small intestinal and proximal and transverse colonic function), (2) by the outflow from the sacral parasympathetic nucleus to the distal colon, and (3) by the splanchnic (sympathetic) innervation of the entire GI tract.

In the most common functional GI disorders, IBS and functional dyspepsia, persistent alterations of autonomic responsiveness are likely to play a role in altered bowel habits, and alterations in gastric emptying, respectively. Evidence for such enhanced responsiveness of autonomic responses in IBS [for review see 1] includes increased responses of distal colonic motility in response to laboratory stress and possibly food intake, and delayed gastric emptying in a subset of patients.

A model of IBS, taking into account altered autonomic regulation of gastric and distal colonic function and based on an upregulation of CRF-containing neurons in Barrington's nucleus (part of the locus coeruleus complex) has recently been reported by Valentino et al. [14]. While descending CRF-containing projections from this pontine nucleus to the distal colon may mediate increased stress and food-induced motor responses of the distal colon, ascending projections to the locus coeruleus and to the forebrain may be responsible for mediating arousal and shifting attention to visceral afferent stimuli. Increased expression of CRF message and release of CRF in IBS patients, or a subset of patients, are also consistent with the reported evidence for certain increased sympathetic responses [23, 24].

Changes in the frequency of high amplitude propagated contraction in the colon, presumably via alterations in vagal colonic regulation, may play an important role in diarrhea [25] and slow transit constipation, thereby determining the predominant bowel habit pattern in IBS [for review see 1]. Thus, while enhanced sacral parasympathetic modulation of the distal colon, reflecting enhanced responsiveness of neurons within the locus coeruleus complex, may be shared by all IBS patients, alterations in vagal output to the small intestine and proximal colon may be variable, depending on severity and the predominant bowel habit.

Neuroendocrine Changes and Mucosal Immune Function

Preliminary evidence for alterations in HPA axis function has been demonstrated in diarrhea-predominant IBS patients who showed decreased 24-hour plasma cortisols, blunted cortisol responses and normal ACTH responses to noxious rectosigmoid distension [26]. In contrast, Heitkemper et al. [27] reported that urine cortisol levels obtained immediately upon rising were significantly higher in a subgroup of IBS women as compared to control women. Even though a thorough characterization of HPA axis responses in patients with functional GI disorders has not been reported, these preliminary findings suggest a pattern of altered glucocorticoid receptor feedback also reported in patients with post-traumatic stress disorder, fibromyalgia and chronic fatigue syndrome.

While it is currently not known if these HPA axis changes are an epiphenomenon, or play a role in the symptom generation and pathophysiology of these syndromes, one may speculate about their possible role (in conjunction with alterations in autonomic gut regulation) in the observed findings in post-infectious IBS patients as well as in unselected IBS patients [28]. The reported persistence of chronic inflammatory mucosal changes after eradication of the infectious organism [29], and increased intestinal permeability and hyperplasia of enterochromaffine cells [30] are consistent with an inadequate physiological response to acute gut inflammation, in particular an inadequate cortisol (and possibly an altered sympathetic) response. Stress-related alterations in cytokine networks, in particular a suppression of cellular immunity and a shift towards humoral immunity (alteration in T helper (Th1)/Th2 balance), have been reported [31]. Multiple reports in the literature on increased intestinal mast cell numbers in IBS patients [32] is consistent with such a Th2 shift.

Changes in Pain Modulation

Following the initial description by Ritchie [33] of increased visceral sensitivity in IBS patients, a large number of laboratories have confirmed the existence of altered visceral perception in IBS [for review see 34, 35]. The current evidence can best be summarized as follows. (1) When tested at baseline and especially when using an ascending series of distensions, IBS patients as a whole show lower discomfort thresholds and greater intensity and unpleasantness ratings during rectal and sigmoid distension. While abnormal perceptual thresholds for discomfort are only seen in about 40–60% of patients, some degree of altered perception as evidenced by a lower discomfort threshold, aberrant referral area, or reproduction of IBS symptoms by balloon distension is seen in nearly all patients [36]. (2) Following a repetitive stimulus, a subset of IBS patients develops profound rectosigmoid hyperalgesia. (3) When exposed to a psychological [37] or physical stressor, such as food intake [38], IBS patients tend to show a greater increase in the subjective ratings of rectosigmoid distension compared to healthy controls. In general, while hypervigilance towards potentially aversive visceral stimuli is present in most IBS patients, alterations in the sensory perception of rectosigmoid distension are most pronounced in female patients with constipation-predominant bowel habit, and nearly absent in male patients with diarrhea-predominant bowel habit [39]. Thus, in human studies, the evidence is strongest for increased vigilance to visceral sensation, as the primary global mechanism of hypersensitivity found in experimental studies is functional GI disorders. Other mechanisms such as increased sensitivity of visceral afferent pathways through central modulation or autonomic dysregulation have also received some but not definitive support across patient subgroups.

There is suggestive evidence for alterations in stress-induced modulation of viscerosomatic sensitivity from human and animal studies. IBS patients show cutaneous normo- or hypoalgesia combined with visceral hypersensitivity [8]. A similar pattern was also seen in a recently described rat IBS model in response to an acute psychological stressor [40]. Preliminary results using psychological laboratory stressors in healthy volunteers suggest a stress-induced increase in colonic or rectosigmoid sensitivity to distension [41]. Even though all published human studies are open to methodological criticism, they are consistent with reported findings in animals of a differential viscerosomatic pain modulation. It is of interest to note that patients with bulimia (who, in contrast to IBS patients, have a hyperactive HPA axis) show cutaneous hypoalgesia as well which precedes symptom exacerbations [42]. Improvement in human sensory testing technologies are needed to better test these mechanisms.

Functional brain imaging studies of IBS patients have shown decreased activation of ventral subdivisions of the anterior cingulate cortex (ACC), and increased activation of the dorsal subdivision [43]. Since dorsal ACC is inhibited by intense visceral stimuli in healthy control subjects (unpublished observations), increased dorsal ACC activation may be related to alterations in attentional processes in IBS in regard to visceral sensory events. Recent evidence suggests that regional brain activation in response to visceral stimulation may differ between male and female IBS patients [44, 45]. While most brain regions showed similar activity patterns between male and female patients, differences were seen primarily in the insular cortex. These observations support the importance of attentional processes in visceral hypersensitivity but also suggest that additional subgroup-specific mechanisms may be important in symptom generation and chronicity.

Conclusions

Distinct activity patterns of the GI tract are linked to the activation of emotion-specific circuits within the brain. Converging evidence suggests an enhanced responsiveness of some of these circuits, in particular those activated in response to a perceived threat and fear, in a subset of IBS patients. This enhanced responsiveness is reflected in greater emotional responses to visceral and emotional stimuli in terms of anger and anxiety, and to an enhanced autonomically mediated modulation of gastric (inhibition) and distal colonic (stimulation) motor and secretory activity. These responses are accompanied by an increased perceptual sensitivity to visceral events. Recent evidence suggests that the enhanced responsiveness can also be observed in response to luminal stressors, such as acute enteric infections. We suggest that the enhanced stress responsiveness discussed in this review may be responsible for the pattern of altered perception, autonomic activity, and pain modulation characteristic for IBS, with some of these mechanisms being more or less important in specific syndrome subgroups.

References

1 Mayer EA: The neurobiology of stress and gastrointestinal disease. Gut 2000;47:861–869.

2 Mayer EA, Naliboff BD, Chang L, Coutinho SV: Stress and irritable bowel syndrome. Am J Physiol Gastrointest Liver Physiol 2001;280: G519–G524.

3 LeDoux JE: The Emotional Brain: The Mysterious Underpinnings of Emotional Life. New York, Simon & Schuster, 1996.

4 Calder AJ, Lawrence AD, Young AW: Neuropsychology of fear and loathing. Nat Rev Neurosci 2001;2:352–363.

5 Mayer EA, Naliboff B, Munakata J: The evolving neurobiology of gut feelings; in Mayer EA, Saper CB (eds): The Biological Basis for Mind Body Interactions. Amsterdam, Elsevier, 2000, pp 195–206.

6 Tache Y, Martinez V, Million M, Rivier J: Corticotropin-releasing factor and the brain-gut motor response to stress. Can J Gastroenterol 1999;13(suppl A):18A–25A.

7 Mayer EA, Craske MG, Naliboff BD: Depression, anxiety and the gastrointestinal system. J Clin Psychiatry 2001;62:28–37.

8 Naliboff BD, Chang L, Munakata J, Mayer EA: Towards an integrative model of irritable bowel syndrome; in Mayer EA, Saper CB (eds): The Biological Basis for Mind Body Interactions. Amsterdam, Elsevier Science, 2000, pp 413–423.

9 Fendt M, Fanselow MS: The neuroanatomical and neurochemical basis of conditioned fear. Neurosci Biobehav Rev 1999;23:743–760.

10 McEwen BS: Protective and damaging effects of stress mediators. N Engl J Med 1998;338: 171–179.

11 Bandler R, Price JL, Keay KA: Brain mediation of active and passive emotional coping; in Mayer EA, Saper CB (eds): The Biological Basis for Mind Body Interactions. Amsterdam, Elsevier Science, 2000, pp 333–349.

12 Vogt BA, Sikes RW, Vogt LJ: Anterior cingulate cortex and the medial pain system; in Vogt BA, Gabriel M (eds): Neurobiology of Cingulate Cortex and Limbic Thalamus: A Comprehensive Handbook. Boston, Birkhäuser, 1993, pp 313–344.

13 Sternberg EM, Chrousos GP, Gold PW: The stress response and the regulation of inflammatory disease. Ann Intern Med 1992;117:854–866.

14 Valentino RJ, Miselis RR, Pavcovich LA: Pontine regulation of pelvic viscera: Pharmacological target for pelvic visceral dysfunction. Trends Pharmacol Sci 1999;20:253–260.

15 Tache Y, Monnikes H, Bonaz B, Rivier J: Role of CRF in stress-related alterations of gastric and colonic motor function. Ann NY Acad Sci 1993;697:233–243.

16 Owens MJ, Nemeroff CB: The role of corticotropin-releasing factor in the pathophysiology of affective and anxiety disorders: Laboratory and clinical studies. Ciba Found Symp 1993; 172:296–316.

17 Timpl P, Spanagel R, Sillaber I, Kresse A, Reul JM, Stalla GK, Blanquet V, Steckler T, Holsboer F, Wurst W: Impaired stress response and reduced anxiety in mice lacking a functional corticotropin-releasing hormone receptor. Nat Genet 1998;19:162–166.

18 Smith GW, Aubry JM, Dellu F, Contarino A, Bilezikjian LM, Gold LH, Chen R, Marchuk Y, Hauser C, Bentley CA, Sawchenko PE, Koob GF, Vale W, Lee KF: Corticotropin-releasing factor receptor 1-deficient mice display decreased anxiety, impaired stress response, and aberrant neuroendocrine development. Neuron 1998;20:1093–1102.

19 Ladd CO, Huot RL, Thrivikraman KV, Nemeroff CB, Meaney MJ, Plotsky P: Long-term behavioral and neuroendocrine adaptations to adverse early experience; in Mayer EA, Saper CB (eds): The Biological Basis for Mind Body Interactions. Amsterdam, Elsevier, 2000, pp 81–103.

20 Fuchs E, Fluegge G: Modulation of binding sites for corticotropin-releasing hormone by chronic psychosocial stress. Psychoneuroendocrinology 1995;20:33–51.

21 Southwick SM, Bremner JD, Rasmusson A, Morgan III CA, Arnsten A, Charney DS: Role of norepinephrine in the pathophysiology and treatment of posttraumatic stress disorder. Biol Psychiatry 1999;46:1192–1204.

22 Sapolsky RM, Krey LC, McEwen BS: Stress down-regulates corticosterone receptors in a site-specific manner in the brain. Endocrinology 1984;114:287–292.

23 Esler MD, Goulston KJ: Levels of anxiety in colonic disorders. N Engl J Med 1973;288:16–20.

24 Jorgensen LS, Bonlokke NJ, Christensen NJ: Life strain, life events, and autonomic response to a psychological stressor in patients with chronic upper abdominal pain. Scand J Gastroenterol 1986;21:605–613.

25 Chey WY, Jin HO, Lee MH, Sun SW, Lee KY: Colonic motility abnormality in patients with irritable bowel syndrome exhibiting abdominal pain and diarrhea. Am J Gastroenterol 2001; 96:1499–1506.

26 Munakata J, Mayer EA, Chang L, Schmulson M, Liu M, Tougas G, Kamath M, Naliboff B: Autonomic and neuroendocrine responses to recto-sigmoid stimulation. Gastroenterology 1998;114:808.

27 Heitkemper M, Jarrett M, Cain K, Shaver J, Bond E, Woods NF, Walker E: Increased urine catecholamines and cortisol in women with irritable bowel syndrome. Am J Gastroenterol 1996;91:906–913.

28 Mayer EA, Collins SM: Evolving pathophysiologic models of functional gastrointestinal disorders. Gastroenterology 2001, in press.

29 Gwee KA: The role of psychological and biological factors in postinfective gut dysfunction. Gut 1999;44:400–406.

30 Spiller RC, Jenkins D, Thornley JP, Hebden JM, Wright T, Skinner M, Neal KR: Increased rectal mucosal enteroendocrine cells, T-lymphocytes, and increased gut permeability following acute *Campylobacter* enteritis and in post-dysenteric irritable bowel syndrome. Gut 2000;47:804–811.

31 Elenkov IJ, Chrousos GP: Stress hormones, Th1/Th2 patterns, pro/anti-inflammatory cytokines and susceptibility to disease. Trends Endocrinol Metab 1999;10:359–368.

32 O'Sullivan M, Clayton N, Breslin NP, Harman I, Bountra C, McLaren A, O'Morain CA: Increased mast cells in the irritable bowel syndrome. Neurogastroenterol Motil 2000;12: 449–457.

33 Ritchie J: Pain from distension of the pelvic colon by inflating a balloon in the irritable colon syndrome. Gut 1973;14:125–132.

34 Naliboff B, Mayer EA: Sensational developments in the irritable bowel. Gut 1996;39:770–771.

35 Whitehead WE, Palsson OS: Is rectal pain sensitivity a biological marker for irritable bowel syndrome: Psychological influences on pain perception. Gastroenterology 1998;115:1263–1271.

36 Mertz H, Naliboff B, Munakata J, Niazi N, Mayer EA: Altered rectal perception is a biological marker of patients with irritable bowel syndrome. Gastroenterology 1995;109:40–52.
37 Dickhaus B, Firooz N, Stains J, Fass R, Mayer EA, Naliboff BD: Psychological stress increases visceral sensitivity in patients with irritable bowel syndrome (IBS) but not controls. Gastroenterology 2001;120:A67.
38 Simrèn M, Abrahamsson H, Björnsson ES: An exaggerated sensory component of the gastrocolonic response in patients with irritable bowel syndrome. Gut 2001;48:20–27.
39 Chang L, Naliboff BD, Schmulson M, Lee OY, Olivas TI, Mayer EA: The role of gender and bowel habit predominance on visceral perception in IBS. Gastroenterology 2001;120:A755.
40 Coutinho SV, Miller JC, Plotsky PM, Mayer EA: Effect of perinatal stress on responses to colorectal distension in adult rats. Soc Neurosci Abstr 1999;25:687.
41 Delvaux MM: Stress and visceral perception. Can J Gastroenterol 1999;13(suppl A):32A–36A.
42 Faris PL, Won Kim S, Meller WH, Goodale RL, Hofbauer RD, Oakman SA, Howard LA, Stevens ER, Eckert ED, Hartman BK: Effect of ondansetron, a 5-HT_3 receptor antagonist, on the dynamic association between bulimic behaviors and pain thresholds. Pain 1998;77:297–304.
43 Naliboff BD, Derbyshire SWG, Munakata J, Berman S, Mandelkern M, Chang L, Mayer EA: Cerebral activation in irritable bowel syndrome patients and control subjects during rectosigmoid stimulation. Psychosom Med 2001;63:365–375.
44 Derbyshire SWG, Naliboff BD, Munakata J, Chang L, Mandelkern M, Berman S, Mayer EA: Gender differences in the central response to visceral pain and anticipation of pain in irritable bowel syndrome (IBS). Gastroenterology 1999;116:A1038.
45 Berman S, Munakata J, Naliboff B, Chang L, Mandelkern M, Silverman DH, Kovalik E, Mayer EA: Gender differences in regional brain response to visceral pressure in IBS patients. Eur J Pain 2000;4:157–172.

Review Article

Digestive Diseases

Dig Dis 2001;19:219–224

Management of Dyspepsia across the Primary-Secondary Healthcare Interface

A. Pali S. Hungin[a] Greg P. Rubin[b]

[a]Centre for Health Studies, University of Durham, and [b]Centre for Primary and Community Care Research, University of Sunderland, UK

Key Words

Dyspepsia · Management · Referral · Guidelines · Primary care · Diagnosis

Abstract

Primary care remains at the frontline of care for most patients and the need to contain healthcare costs has led to a re-evaluation of the divide between primary and secondary care. Dyspepsia has a community prevalence of 25–50%, and forms 5% of the primary care physician's workload, 10% of whom are referred to a specialist. Problems presenting in primary care tend to be undifferentiated; those who do not have alarm symptoms and are under the age of 55 years are unlikely to have serious pathology. Management is largely symptom driven, on an empirical basis rather than on a diagnostic model as in secondary care where investigation rates are higher. The predictive value of symptoms for a specific diagnosis is small; primary care physicians include gastro-oesophageal reflux disease as part of the dyspepsia complex and the overall expenditure on acid suppression therapy is relatively large. The availability of open-access investigations such as endoscopy has influenced specialist referral rates and the ability to diagnose and treat patients with *Helicobacter pylori*-related problems has opened further opportunities. However, variations in the availability of the recommended diagnostic tests and the implications to primary care clinical practice of some of the new management recommendations (Maastricht II) in some national settings illustrate the divide with secondary care. The gap between primary and secondary care is narrowing in gastroenterology and the two groups need to continue collaboration to attain effective and cost-effective management for their patients.

Introduction

Although health structures vary, primary care remains at the forefront of care for most patients in Western Europe [1] and increasingly in the USA. Patients often present with problems that are largely of an undifferentiated nature. The predominant role of the primary care physician is to separate problems that require action from that which do not. The presenting problems during some consultations may be undifferentiated to the extent that they defy the identification of the systems involved; in other cases, multi-system involvement with complex problems, e.g. impaired mobility due to arthritis as well as dyspepsia, requires a carefully considered approach.

In primary care, the clinician's role is to ensure that a serious problem is not overlooked and to 'ensure normali-

KARGER

Fax + 41 61 306 12 34
E-Mail karger@karger.ch
www.karger.com

0257–2753/01/0193–0219$17.50/0

Accessible online at:
www.karger.com/journals/ddi

Prof. A. Pali S. Hungin, MBBS, MD, FRCGP
Professor of Primary Care and General Practice
Centre for Health Studies, University of Durham
32 Old Elvet, Durham DH1 3HN (UK)
Tel. +44 1642 789026, Fax +44 1642 791629, E-Mail a.p.s.hungin@durham.ac.uk

ty'. In contrast, the secondary care physician, particularly in a setting where patients are referred from primary care, has the traditional remit of confirming a diagnosis and instituting appropriate care. This has been described as 'marginalizing uncertainty'. In settings where the specialist is directly consulted by the patient, i.e. without referral from a primary care physician, a degree of selection will have occurred based on the patient's perception of the nature of their problem. Unless there is a major doubt it is likely that the specialist will consider investigations relevant to that speciality, an approach which differs from primary care. Whilst primary care physicians tend to work 'longitudinally', i.e. by using time and repeated consultations as a management tool, specialists are more likely to attempt a definitive diagnosis expediently following the initial consultation. This will be reflected in investigation rates and, invariably, costs.

Despite these fundamental differences between primary and secondary care in the way in which patients' problems are delineated and managed, the gap between primary and secondary care is probably narrower in gastroenterology than in other specialities. There are a number of reasons for this: the development of accurate diagnostic investigations (notably endoscopy and ultrasonography) which have become increasingly available to primary care physicians, the development of acceptable and effective *Helicobacter pylori* eradication therapies, and the advent of powerful drugs such as H2 receptor blockers and proton pump inhibitors (PPIs) for use in acid-sensitive disorders. As a result, *H. pylori*-related diseases and acid-sensitive disorders can be effectively managed in primary care, though, paradoxically, the high cost to healthcare systems of therapies such as PPIs relates in large part to their extensive use in primary care.

Dyspepsia: Prevalence, Workload and Resource Implications

Dyspepsia is a common problem. The prevalence of dyspepsia in the community is between 25 and 50% [2–5], and in the UK 2% of the population consult a general practitioner (GP)/family practitioner (FP) with a new or first episode of dyspepsia each year [6]. Approximately 10% of the workload of a GP is in gastroenterology of which 50% is related to the upper gastrointestinal tract [6]. In the UK (population 55 million), 280,000 endoscopies were performed in 1995 at a cost of GBP 70 million, and GBP 450 million was spent on acid suppression drugs alone [7]. Up to 1% of the population of the UK is thought to be taking prescribed medication for dyspepsia at any one time [8] with those on long term PPIs constituting a large proportion of this group [9]. It is likely that these figures are higher in many other western countries, especially in the USA where more investigations are performed than in Europe.

Despite the high prevalence of dyspepsia in the community, less than 50% of sufferers consult their GP/FP [10, 11]. The reasons for consulting are less related to the severity or duration of symptoms than to perceptions of the potential consequences of the symptoms. These factors include a fear of cardiac problems, cancer or a family history of ulcer disease [10–12].

The Interpretation of Dyspepsia: Variations between Primary and Secondary Care

The current academic definition of dyspepsia, as described by the Rome II consensus, is 'pain or discomfort centred in the upper abdomen' [13]. For most GPs/FPs, reflux disease is an integral part of 'dyspepsia', reflecting the everyday pragmatic need to categorize this problem [14]. This is supported by the Canadian Dyspepsia Working Group Guidelines which focused on the conceptual framework that primary care physicians follow when a patient presents with uninvestigated dyspeptic symptoms [14]. The Rome II criteria further describe functional dyspepsia as a problem which has been present for 12 or more weeks in the previous year and where organic lesions have been excluded by investigation; two subgroups are defined, based on ulcer-like and dysmotility-like predominant symptoms. Although appropriate for research and categorization these definitions are removed from management in pragmatic clinical care.

The Roles of GPs/FPs and Specialists

The 1991 World Organization of Family Physicians defined the GP/FP as a clinician who provided comprehensive care to every individual seeking medical care and arranged for other health personnel to provide services where necessary [15, 16]. The requirements for being a GP/FP include (a) the provision of comprehensive care – not only curative but also in relation to rehabilitation, prevention and health promotion (b) the co-ordination of healthcare, including a responsibility to make available to patients the differing resources of healthcare and (c) resource management.

Table 1. Potential advantages of a shared care approach (from Travis et al. [17])

Patients
Greater continuity of treatment and follow-up
Easier access to local medical advice
Reduced hospital visits
Shorter waiting times
Greater contact with a doctor who is more aware of their social and family circumstances
Family physicians
Patients may be more open with doctors with whom they are familiar
Opportunity to provide better patient care
Development of new skills and broader knowledge in gastroenterology
Stronger relations with specialists
Reduced costs from more selective referral and follow-up
Specialists
Encourages referrals appropriate for specialist care
Reduced clinic size owing to fewer follow-ups
More time available for patients requiring specialist management
Opportunity to provide better patient care
Stronger relations with family physicians
Reduced costs by more selective follow-up

Resource management has particular implications for the way patients are managed throughout the western economies. The need to contain rising healthcare costs has led to a new remit for primary care, as a filter and as a focus for overall healthcare. The concept of managed care, with its objectives of quality and continuity of care, together with cost effectiveness and cost containment, has led to the traditional primary-secondary care divide being viewed in a new light. This is illustrated by changes in care structures in the USA through the emergence of Health Maintenance Organizations, and in the UK, attempts to integrate care through Primary Care Organizations and their hospital and social care counterparts. Increasingly, these initiatives include shared management with regulated and combined prescribing policies (table 1).

Influences on the Primary Care Management of Dyspepsia and Specialist Referral

A major influence on the management of patients with dyspepsia is the structure of the local healthcare system [18]. Where there is an established primary care structure and a formal referral system (e.g. the UK, Netherlands and Denmark) the approach will differ from those countries where patients have direct access to a specialist (e.g. Germany, France and Italy). In the latter group, management is more likely to be associated with investigation rather than empirical treatment as in primary care.

In primary care the risk of serious life-threatening lesions is low in the undifferentiated population presenting with dyspepsia. The majority of dyspeptic patients can be managed on a symptomatic basis, without necessarily the diagnosis of a specific lesion, either with lifestyle advice or with drugs aimed at symptom control [19]. A specific diagnosis is likely to require further investigations, particularly endoscopy, and avoiding these significantly contains healthcare costs.

The management of dyspepsia across both primary and secondary care has also been influenced by the changing trends in pathology. In most western countries, peptic ulcer rates have declined whilst the prevalence of gastro-oesophageal reflux disease (GERD) has risen. In the UK, peptic ulcers are detected in less than 5% of endoscopies whilst GERD is diagnosed in more than 25%. On the basis that peptic ulcers and cancer are unlikely in the younger patient, there is a trend towards avoiding endoscopy in this group [20].

The possibility of cancer, a driver for investigation and referral, remains less than 2% in endoscopic series [21]; alarm symptoms and increasing age are associated with organic lesions, although these are associated with relatively advanced disease [22, 23]. Whist the earlier detection of gastric cancer may lead to a better prognosis [24, 25], evidence also suggests that acid suppression therapy may be associated with a delay in the diagnosis of cancer [26].

These data present a confusing picture in terms of the appropriateness of referral for investigation or specialist management of patients with dyspepsia. There is universal acceptance of the need for investigating patients with alarm symptoms but the situation is less clear in the remainder. Patients who are not at high risk and respond to acid suppression therapy are likely to have GERD and could be managed in primary care alone. As some of these patients will require long-term therapy it has been argued that they should have an investigation at some stage, in part to establish if they might have Barrett's oesophagus, a potentially pre-malignant condition. Those who do not respond to empirical therapy are more likely to be referred for investigation or for a specialist opinion – invariably, the majority will have no detectable lesions and are unlikely to benefit from any specific interventions, although a subgroup, amounting to 1 in 15 of those who have *H. pylori* infection, will benefit from eradication therapy [27].

The rate of referral to specialists in those countries which have structured primary care is relatively low at around 10% [28]. Rates of referral are likely to be influenced by the availability of open-access investigative services, which allow the primary care physician greater control over patient management, and the funding mechanisms for tests, investigations and drugs. These factors can also influence the local capacity to implement best practice guidelines [29].

Do All Patients Need Investigation or Referral for a Definitive Diagnosis?

Serious causes for dyspepsia are rare in patients without alarm symptoms and in those under the age of 55 years. Nevertheless, the positive predictive value of symptoms is poor [30–32] and the clinical diagnosis is further confounded by the overlap of symptoms from upper and lower gastrointestinal lesions, particularly irritable bowel syndrome [12, 30, 31, 33, 34]. The positive predictive value of a clinical diagnosis of GERD is relatively high [35], however, and can be enhanced using a structured questionnaire [36] or a diagnostic acid suppression test [37]. As most patients presenting with upper gastrointestinal symptoms are likely to have reflux and will respond to empirical acid suppression therapy, the need to attain an exact diagnosis in otherwise well patients is debatable.

Even using endoscopy, a definitive diagnosis is made in a minority of patients (30–40%), essentially in those with GERD or peptic ulcers. The availability of open-access gastroscopy in the UK has had no impact on the median time from presentation to the first diagnosis of gastric cancer. The diagnostic yield rises with the use of ultrasonography and pH monitoring, although the latter is used only in a fraction of patients, largely those in whom this is a diagnostic necessity because of management difficulties. In some patients there might be the need to eliminate the possibility of Barrett's oesophagitis. Many, however, may need investigation or referral for reasons of reassurance and the clinician's course of action should always be sensitive to the individual patient's circumstances and health beliefs.

Dyspepsia and *H. pylori* Management Guidelines – Opportunities and Problems

There is a host of published and in-preparation guidelines in this field; for the sake of illustration only three are discussed.

The Canadian Dyspepsia Working Group Guidelines for Uninvestigated Dyspepsia [14]

These have the advantage of having a strong primary care base, using a pragmatic definition of dyspepsia which includes GERD. They utilize the following decision steps in formulating a management approach: (a) that the symptoms originate in the upper gastrointestinal tract; (b) the presence of alarm features; (c) the use of nonsteroidal and inflammatory drugs; (d) the presence of dominant reflux symptoms, and (e) evidence for *H. pylori* infection.

It is recommended that all patients over the age of 50 years who present with new onset dyspepsia and those who present with alarm features should receive prompt investigation, preferably by endoscopy. The implication is that if the GP/FP does not have open-access investigative services, the patient should be referred. Those with uninvestigated dyspepsia who use NSAIDs regularly should cease NSAID therapy to enable assessment, treatment with NSAID prophylaxis or for referral for investigation. The guidelines reiterate that reflux disease can be diagnosed on clinical grounds if the dominant symptoms are heartburn or regurgitation and that acid suppression therapy is appropriate. In other patients, *H. pylori* testing is recommended with eradication therapy for those positive. Those with a negative result should have their symptoms treated with optimal antisecretory therapy.

The European Society for Primary Care Gastroenterology Guidelines ('The Management of H. pylori *Infection in Primary Care') [29]*

The basis of these guidelines is a recognition of the variation of practice and conditions in different countries. These variations include differing healthcare systems, economic circumstances, the availability of drugs, investigations and the resistance rates to antimicrobials. Beyond providing a basic template, the guidelines recommend adaptation of action to suit local circumstances. The following main recommendations are made: (a) Patients with alarm symptoms and older patients with their first onset of dyspepsia should have a prompt endoscopic investigation to establish a diagnosis. (b) Patients with a new diagnosis of duodenal or gastric ulcer and those with a previously diagnosed ulcer who become symptomatic, or are taking long-term antisecretory therapy, should receive eradication therapy. (c) *H. pylori* testing should be considered for those who consult with recurrent symptoms of dyspepsia, either as part of a test and treat or a test plus endoscopy strategy. (d) *H. pylori* testing in eradication is not recommended for patients with non-ulcer dyspepsia or for the family members of *H. pylori*-infected patients.

The Maastricht II Guidelines

These provide comprehensive advice on dyspepsia management in relation to *H. pylori* infection. In addition to recommending eradication in peptic ulcer disease, the guidelines endorse a test and treat strategy in younger patients, in primary care. However, they contain a number of items which primary care physicians are likely to find contentious. Amongst these is the suggestion that patients likely to require long-term PPI therapy should have *H. pylori* testing and eradication, and that, on the basis of reducing the incidence of prior peptic ulcers, those commencing NSAID therapy should also have *H. pylori* eradication if are positive. This advice has far-reaching workload and economic consequences in primary care and is regarded by many as contentious. The guidelines also recommend the Urea Breath Test or the Stool Antigen Test as the optimal tests for *H. pylori* detection; since these are not widely available in primary care, the policy also has referral implications.

Conclusions

Dyspepsia lends itself to seamless management across the primary-secondary care divide, the boundaries between which are increasingly dissolving in gastroenterology. This is because of the evolution of dyspepsia management due to the advent of powerful acid suppression drugs, accurate investigations such as endoscopy and an understanding of the role of *H. pylori.* Most patients can be managed in either primary or secondary care but there are significant differences in approach; in primary care the management of those not at risk of serious lesions is likely to be symptom-based, whilst in secondary care the need for a definitive diagnosis remains paramount. In patients whose investigations do not reveal a cause of the dyspepsia, management remains a problem – whilst a small proportion of those who are *H. pylori*-positive may benefit from eradication therapy, the rest represent a challenge for both the primary and secondary care physician. If fully worked up from primary care and referred, these patients represent a particular difficulty for the secondary care physician.

Although guidelines exist for the management of patients with dyspepsia, it is important that they should be contextualized for local conditions. Some guideline recommendations, notably some of the advice in the Maastricht II guidelines, sit uneasily within the context and resource availability of primary care and may cause tensions between primary and secondary care clinicians. The effective, timely and cost-effective management of dyspepsia requires close collaboration and understanding between primary and secondary care clinicians.

References

1 Boerma WGW, Fleming DM: The Role of General Practice in Primary Health Care. WHO. London, The Stationery Office, 1998.
2 Knill-Jones RP: Geographical differences in the prevalence of dyspepsia. Scand J Gastroenterol 1991;26(suppl 182):17–24.
3 Jones R, Lydeard S: Dyspepsia in the community: A follow up study. Br J Clin Pract 1992; 48:95–97.
4 Penston JG, Pounder RE: A survey of dyspepsia in Great Britain. Aliment Pharmacol Ther 1996;10:83–89.
5 Jones RH, Lydeard SE, Hobbs FDR, et al: Dyspepsia in England and Scotland. Gut 1990;31: 401–405.
6 McCormick A, Fleming D, Charlton J: Morbidity Statistics from General Practice: Fourth National Study 1991–92. London, Office of Population Censuses and Surveys, 1995.
7 Statistics of Prescriptions Dispensed in the Family Health Services Authorities: England 1984–94. Statistical Bulletin. London, HMSO, 1995.
8 Ryder SD, O'Reilly S, Miller RJ, et al: Long-term acid suppression treatment in general practice. BMJ 1994;308:827–830.
9 Hungin APS, Rubin GP, O'Flanagan H: Long-term prescribing of proton pump inhibitors in general practice. Br J Gen Pract 1999;49:451–453.
10 Lydeard S, Jones R: Factors affecting the decision to consult with dyspepsia: Comparison of consulters and non-consulters. J R Coll Gen Pract 1989;39:495–498.
11 Holtmann G, Goebell H, Talley NJ: Dyspepsia in consulters and non-consulters: Prevalence, health-seeking behaviour and risk factors. Eur J Gastroenterol Hepatol 1994;6:917–924.
12 Talley NJ, Zinsmeister AR, Schleck CD, Melton LJ III: Dyspepsia and dyspepsia subgroups: A population-based study. Gastroenterology 1992;102:1259–1268.
13 Talley NJ, Stanghellini V, Heading R, et al: Functional gastroduodenal disorders. Gut 1999;45(suppl 2):137–142.
14 Veldhuyzen van Zanten SJO, Flook N, et al: An evidence-based approach to the management of uninvestigated dyspepsia in the era of *Helicobacter pylori.* Can Med Assoc J 2000; 162(suppl 12):S1–S23.
15 WONCA 1991: The Role of the General Practitioner/Family Physician in Health Care Systems. A Statement from the World Organisation of National Colleges, Academies and Academic Associations of General Practitioners/ Family Physicians. Victoria, WONCA, 1991.
16 LHV (Dutch Medical Association of General Practitioners): Basic Job Description of the General Practitioner. Utrecht, LHV, 1993.
17 Travis S, Stevens R, Dalton H: Shared Care in Gastroenterology, Oxford, Isis Medical, 1997.
18 De Wit NJ, Mendive J, Seifert B, Cardin F, Rubin G: Guidelines on the management of *H. pylori* in primary care: Development of an implementation strategy. Family Pract 2000; 17(suppl 2):S27–S32.
19 Meineche-Schmidt V, Rubin G, de Wit NJ: *Helicobacter pylori* infection: A comparative review of existing management guidelines. Family Pract 2000;17(suppl 2):S2–S5.

20 Dyspepsia Management Guidelines: Guidelines in Gastroenterology. British Society for Gastroenterology, London, BSG, 1996.
21 American Gastroenterological Association (AGA) Clinical Practice and Practice Economics Committee: Evaluation of Dyspepsia. Bethesda, AGA, 1998, vol 114, pp 582–595.
22 Adang RP, Vismans JF, Talmon JL, et al: Appropriateness of indications for diagnostic upper gastrointestinal endoscopy: Association with relevant endoscopic disease. Gastrointest Endosc 1995;42:390–397.
23 Williams B, Luckas M, Ellington JHM, et al: Do young patients with dyspepsia need investigation? Lancet 1998;ii:149–151.
24 Sue-Ling HM, Johnston D, Martin IG, et al: Gastric cancer: A curable disease in Britain. BMJ 1993;307:591–596.
25 Hallissey MT, Allum WH, Jewkes AG, et al: Early detection of gastric cancer. BMJ 1990; 301:513–515.
26 Bramble MG, Suvokovic Z, Hungin APS: Detection of upper gastrointestinal cancer in patients taking anti-secretory therapy prior to endoscopy. Gut 2000;46:464–467.
27 Moayyedi P, Soo S, Deeks J, et al: Systematic review and economic evaluation of *Helicobacter pylori* eradication treatment for non-ulcer dyspepsia. BMJ 2000;321:659–664.
28 Hungin APS, Bramble MG, O'Callaghan H: Reasons for variations in the use of open access gastroscopy by general practitioners. Gut 1995; 36:180–182.
29 Rubin G (ed): The management of *H. pylori* infection in primary care. Family Pract 2000(suppl 2):S1–S35.
30 Johannessen T, Peterson H, Kleveland PM, et al: The predictive value of history in dyspepsia. Scand J Gastroenterol 1990;25:689–697.
31 Talley NJ, Weaver AL, Tesmer DL, et al: Lack of discriminant value of dyspepsia sub-groups in patients referred for upper endoscopy. Gastroenterology 1993;105:1378–1386.
32 Bytzer P, Hansen JM, Havelund T, et al: Predicting endoscopic diagnosis in the dyspeptic patient: The value of clinical judgement. Eur J Gastroenterol Hepatol 1996;8:359–363.
33 Agreus L, Svardsudd K, Nyren O, et al: Irritable bowel syndrome and dyspepsia in the general population: Overlap and lack of stability over time. Gastroenterology 1995;109:671–680.
34 Grainger SL, Klass HJ, Rake MO, et al: Prevalence of dyspepsia: The epidemiology of overlapping symptoms. Postgrad Med J 1994;70: 154–161.
35 Klauser AG, Schindlebeck NE, Muller-Lissner SA: Symptoms in gastro-oesophageal reflux disease. Lancet 1990;335:205–208.
36 Carlsson R, Dent J, Bolling-Sternevald, et al: The usefulness of a structured questionnaire in the assessment of symptomatic gastro-oesophageal reflux disease. Scand J Gastroenterol 1998;33:1023–1029.
37 Fass R, Ofman JJ, Sampliner RE, Camargo L, Wendel C, Fennerty MB: The omeprazole test is as sensitive as 24-hour oesophageal pH monitoring in diagnosing gastro-oesophageal reflux disease in symptomatic patients with erosive oesophagitis. Aliment Pharmacol Ther 2000; 14:389–396.

Review Article

Digestive Diseases

Dig Dis 2001;19:225–231

How Valuable Is the Application on Consensus Guidelines in the Management of Functional Gastrointestinal Disorders?

D. Vaira[a] L. Gatta[a] C. Ricci[a] L. D'Anna[b] M. Miglioli[a]

[a]1st Medical Clinic, S. Orsola Hospital, University of Bologna, and [b]Gastrointestinal Unit, Main Army Hospital, Rome, Italy

Key Words
Guidelines · Rome II criteria · Symptoms · Functional dyspepsia · Irritable bowel disease

Abstract
When patients complain of problems, physicians are used to look for some physical or physiological abnormality ruling out infections, inflammatory or cancer. Unfortunately, when we talk about functional disorders we usually cannot observe any defects and it is only possible for us to know of them through the words of our patients. Developing criteria and guidelines is not an easy process, in particular for functional gastrointestinal diseases, when no disease-based biological markers exist. It is difficult to define a medical disorder in the absence of a biological 'gold standard'. The Rome II classification is based on the assumption that for each disorder there are symptom custers. Symptoms have in common disturbances in sensory and/or motor gastrointestinal function, which sometimes may overlap across anatomic regions. Nevertheless, several studies provide evidence for site-specific syndromes.

'A good set of bowels is worth more to a man than any quantity of brains'

Introduction

This statement by Josh Billings (1818–1885) recognises what physicians have seen in their practices for centuries. It is quite common for people to be affected by gastrointestinal problems producing symptoms of pain, nausea, vomiting, bloating, diarrhoea, constipation, difficult passage of food or faeces, or any combination [1]. Indeed we have many references to gut abnormalities in ancient and early European literature. One of the first descriptions of irritable bowel syndrome (IBS) dates back to 1818 and it points attention to three cardinal symptoms: abdominal pain, 'derangement of ... digestion and flatulence' [2]. In 1849 Cumming [3] incredulously reported that there were patients in whom the bowels were at one time constipated, at another lax. Unfortunately this enigma is still present!

Medical diagnosis generally requires the observation of anatomical or physiological abnormalities, and the description of diseases as well as criteria for diagnosis follow quite naturally. When patients complain of problems,

KARGER

Fax + 41 61 306 12 34
E-Mail karger@karger.ch
www.karger.com

0257–2753/01/0193–0225$17.50/0

Accessible online at:
www.karger.com/journals/ddi

Prof. Dino Vaira
1st Medical Clinic, S. Orsola Hospital
Nuove Patologie, Via Massarenti 9
I–40138 Bologna (Italy)
Tel. +39 051 6364140, Fax +39 051 398794, E-Mail vairadin@med.unibo.it

physicians are used to looking for some physical or physiological abnormality ruling out infections, inflammation or cancer. Unfortunately when we talk about functional disorders these processes are not possible. We usually cannot observe any defect and it is only possible for us to know about these disorders through the words of our patients. As more than half of the gut disorders encountered by physicians in primary care and gastroenterologists are functional, we should try to understand the pathophysiological mechanisms which determine these symptoms and to develop methods which allow us to recognise and diagnose them [4].

Indeed it is still common in medical practice when no organic abnormalities are found to label the patient as having 'functional symptoms' and treat him/her symptomatically [5]. But how often do we use this label correctly?

Needs for Guidelines

For too long, functional gastrointestinal disorders (FGDs) have been described by what they are not, rather than as real entities, despite being real enough for the patients. Furthermore too often these patients are considered as 'psychogenic' or 'neurogenic'. Until recently, limited knowledge about the pathophysiology of the FGDs and the need to exclude 'organic' disease for a diagnosis has led physicians to feel uncertain about the legitimacy of these symptoms as genuine disorders [6]. Moreover, some physicians do not 'feel confident' to manage patients with these conditions and might even avoid caring for patients with these problems. However, over the past two decades something has changed and now these conditions have been legitimised and increased attention is being given to this field. Indeed there has been a shift in conceptualising these disorders from a disease-based, reductionistic model, where effort is directed toward identifying a single underlying biological aetiology, to a more integrated biopsychosocial model of illness [7, 8]. This new model enables the understanding of the symptoms as physiologically multi-determined (i.e. altered motility, brain-gut disregulation) and as modifiable by socio-cultural and psychosocial influences.

There has also been an improvement in investigative techniques which seem able to support the new understanding of brain-gut interactions. Improved motility assessment, development of barostat, imaging of the brain (positron emission topography), and functional magnetic resonance imaging have led to a larger number of international meetings about FGDs and an increasing effort by pharmaceutical companies to identify how to diagnose and treat patients with these disorders.

Thompson [9] made the first attempt to classify all the FGDs. In the 1990s the first Rome criteria was proposed which classified functional gastrointestinal syndromes into 21 entities in five anatomical regions of the gut [10]. Following this, in 1999 there was the publication of the Rome II criteria (table 1).

Developing criteria and guidelines is not an easy process, in particular for FGDs. Probably these disorders are one of the 'grey zones' of modern medicine. There is a dilemma as to how to make a diagnosis when no disease-based biological markers exist. It is difficult to define a medical disorder in the absence of a biological 'gold standard'. As a consequence there is also the problem of how to identify patients for clinical trials and other research studies. It is not possible to define FGDs by exclusion because this leads to heterogeneous groups that cannot be compared among studies.

The Rome II classification is based on the assumption that for each disorder there are symptom clusters which 'breed true' across clinical and population groups [11]. The rationale for classifying the FGDs into symptom-based subgroups has three bases: site-specific differences; epidemiological data, and the need for diagnostic standards of clinical care and research [12].

Patients complaining of FGDs report a wide variety of symptoms affecting different regions. Symptoms have in common disturbances in sensory and/or motor gastrointestinal function, which sometimes may overlap across anatomic regions. Nevertheless several studies provide evidence for site-specific syndromes [13]. Interestingly epidemiologic studies show that these conditions have a similar prevalence in different studies and populations. Frequencies of bowel symptom patterns reported from England, France and China are nearly identical. The last point is quite important. We know that, by definition, the physiological features of diagnostic value are not present in FGDs. As the patients come to the physician with their symptoms, the use of a symptom-based classification system is rational.

Symptom-based criteria are being more frequently used in medicine. Indeed they are used in psychiatry (e.g. DSM-IV) [14] and rheumatology [15], and are becoming accepted in gastroenterology. Symptom-based criteria can help in the diagnosis and treatment, thereby also reducing unnecessary diagnostic tests. The Rome II criteria are classified by anatomical region: oesophageal, gastroduodenal, bowel and functional abdominal pain, biliary and

Table 1. Functional gastrointestinal disorders

Esophageal disorders
Globus
Rumination syndrome
Functional chest pain of presumed esophageal origin
Functional heartburn
Functional dysphagia
Nonspecified functional esophageal disorder
Gastroduodenal disorders
Functional dyspepsia
Ulcer-like dyspepsia
Dysmotility-like dyspepsia
Unspecified (nonspecific) dyspepsia
Aerophagia
Functional vomiting
Bowel disorders
Irritable bowel syndrome
Functional abdominal bloating
Functional constipation
Functional diarrhea
Nonspecified functional bowel disorder
Functional abdominal pain
Functional abdominal pain syndrome
Nonspecified functional abdominal pain
Biliary disorders
Gallbladder dysfunction
Sphincter of Oddi dysfunction
Anorectal disorders
Functional fecal incontinence
Functional anorectal pain
Levator ani syndrome
Proctalgia fugax
Pelvic floor dyssynergia
Functional pediatric disorders
Vomiting
Infant regurgitation
Infant rumination syndrome
Cyclic vomiting syndrome
Abdominal pain
Functional dyspepsia
Irritable bowel syndrome
Functional abdominal pain
Abdominal migraine
Aerophagia
Functional diarrhea
Disorders of defecation
Infant dyschezia
Functional constipation
Functional fecal retention
Nonretentive fecal soiling

anorectal. For each region we have a definition, epidemiology, clinical evaluation, physiologic features, psychologic features and treatment of the different FGDs.

If there has been some modification in the criteria since Rome I, this is justified. However, it is important to keep in mind some important points. It is possible, due to the high frequency of the FGDs, that there is a coexistence with other organic diseases. Inflammatory bowel diseases and irritable bowel syndrome (IBS) seem to have a strong association [16]. Similarly *Helicobacter pylori* infection needs to be excluded and/or treated in patients with functional dyspepsia. It is also important to remember that different FGDs may coexist. If criteria for IBS and functional dyspepsia are fulfilled, both the diagnoses coexist.

Another important point is that to make a diagnosis, symptoms should be present for at least 12 months out of the previous year. This is a change from the former criteria, which only required symptoms to be present in the previous 3 months. The reason for this change is that symptoms might not have been present in the previous 3 months, but may have been present prior to that time. Indeed the 12 weeks need to be consecutive, and within each week, symptoms are only required for 1 of 7 days. However, there are some exceptions, for example chronic functional abdominal pain requires 6 months of symptoms.

Rome II Guidelines: Are They Useful?

A nation-wide cross-sectional survey in order to collect information on practice demographics and types of diagnoses was performed in 1997 in the USA. 376 of 767 American Gastroenterological Association (AGA) members selected randomly from the AGA directory [17] returned their surveys. Despite changes in health care, functional disorders remained the most common group of disorders seen in gastroenterology practices. Indeed, IBS was reported as the most common disorder (19%). As a group FGDs (IBS, non-ulcer dyspepsia, and other functional disorders) were by far the most common (35%).

Clearly it is important to have valid guidelines. The Rome II criteria are probably the best known since they have been published with important consequences. First of all, more gastroenterologists and more physicians than before know that there are criteria and guidelines for FGDs. These guidelines are the work of a wide panel of experts trying to create a 'standardised language' particularly in terms of definitions and clinical evaluation. For example considering functional oesophageal disorders, it

Table 2. Rome II diagnostic criteria for functional dyspepsia

At least 12 weeks, which need not be consecutive, within the preceding 12 months of:

1 Persistent or recurrent dyspepsia (pain or discomfort centered in the upper abdomen)

2 No evidence of organic disease (including at upper endoscopy) that is likely to explain the symptoms

3 No evidence that dyspepsia is exclusively relieved by defecation or associated with the onset of a change in stool frequency or stool form (i.e., not irritable bowel)

is stressed that the criteria for diagnosis rest not only on compatible symptoms but also on the exclusion of structural, metabolic, pathology-based motor disorders (e.g. achalasia) and pathological reflux (evidence of reflux oesophagitis on endoscopy or abnormal acid exposure time during ambulatory oesophageal pH monitoring) [18]. Thus, it should now be clear that before talking about functional heartburn or dysphagia it is mandatory to rule out some more common diseases. Consideration of functional dyspepsia and IBS (the two most common causes of FGDs) are more intriguing but also more complex.

Functional Dyspepsia

Dyspepsia is a common condition affecting approximately 30% of the population in industrialised countries. It can be caused by various organic, systemic and metabolic diseases, but in about 50% of patients no clear cause is found, hence the term 'functional' dyspepsia [19]. Thus the diagnosis assumes that the patient has been fully investigated ruling out organic diseases, such as peptic ulcer, gastro-oesophageal reflux disease (GORD) and gastric cancer, and also has no apparent structural pathophysiologic or microbiologic abnormalities.

According to the Rome II criteria functional dyspepsia refers to pain or discomfort centred in the upper abdomen (table 2). This implies that the pain or discomfort is mainly in or around the midline. Thus pain in the right or left hypocondrium is not considered to be representative of dyspepsia. Moreover, from an aetiological viewpoint, these patients can be divided further into 3 subgroups: 'ulcer-like dyspepsia', i.e. patients reporting pain centred in the upper abdomen as the predominant or most severe symptom; 'dysmotility-like dyspepsia', i.e. patients mainly reporting discomfort centred in the upper abdomen, and 'unspecified dyspepsia', i.e. symptomatic patients whose symptoms do not fulfil the criteria for ulcer-like or dysmotility-like dyspepsia. A reflux-like subgroup is not present in the Rome II criteria because patients with predominant heartburn are considered to have symptomatic GORD. However, it is noted that some patients with functional dyspepsia may have heartburn as an additional symptom, secondary to abdominal pain or discomfort.

So we can have patients complaining of pain or discomfort; but what does discomfort mean exactly? This 'word' used in the Rome II criteria could be a potential linguistic problem because it is a typical English expression which is difficult to translate. Discomfort is used to refer to a subjective, negative feeling that the patient does not interpret as pain and which, if fully assessed, can include a number of specific symptoms like early satiety, fullness, bloating in the upper abdomen and nausea. However, this distinction is not universally accepted because it should be possible to consider discomfort as a mild form of pain [20]. Nevertheless, it is well recognised that nociceptive and non-nociceptive afferent fibres, involved in the transmission of different types of visceral stimuli to the central nervous system, are distinguishable. Thus, post-prandial fullness, nausea, and vomiting can be severe without being painful [21].

Some studies have tried to focus on whether the identification of predominant symptoms, as implicitly suggested by the Rome II criteria, can improve the diagnosis and management of functional dyspepsia. Indeed the utility of this approach has been found to be reliable in GORD where it is possible to diagnose and manage patients on the basis of the presence and severity of the predominant symptom [22].

In a recent study 483 patients with chronic functional dyspepsia were assessed in order to investigate the relationship between symptom severity, demographic features and gastric dysmotility [23]. In particular the authors looked at the two main symptoms on which Rome II criteria focus attention: epigastric pain and discomfort. They found that it was possible to recognise predominant symptoms in nearly two thirds of the patients. Indeed their first group was characterised by predominant epigastric pain, male gender (61%) with a higher than ideal body weight and normal gastric emptying, and the second group was characterised by predominant discomfort, female gender (60%) with lower than ideal body weight, a high frequency of associated IBS (30%) and delayed gastric emptying (42%). A third group (about one third of the patients) did not show any predominant symptoms.

Talley et al. [24] conducted two large trials to evaluate whether sub-groups of dyspepsia, based on ranking of the most bothersome complaint, would identify responders to acid suppression with proton pump inhibitors. It was found that patients complaining of pain and heartburn and/or regurgitation had significantly greater symptom relief with proton pump inhibitors when compared with patients with dysmotility-like symptoms. Thus, predominant symptoms may be useful in predicting the response to treatment.

However, as for other FGDs, we can only improve diagnosis and treatment in functional dyspepsia if we are able to properly assess the subjective perceptions of patients. Carlsson et al. [22] tested two validated questionnaires to evaluate patients with suspected GORD or functional dyspepsia. The former used simple descriptive language whilst the latter used standard language. Interestingly only 32% of patients who reported the sensation of heartburn in the simple one did so in the standard one. This underlines the necessity of using simple but validated instruments to understand symptoms and improve knowledge about these problems.

Irritable Bowel Syndrome

Surveys of Western populations have revealed inflammatory bowel disease in 15–20% of adolescents and adults, with a higher prevalence in women. IBS has a chronic relapsing course and overlaps with other FGDs. There is increasing attention on IBS. The results of a Medline literature search for IBS by decade for the 30 years ending with 1997 show that the number of articles published rose from 51 between 1968 and 1977 to 893 between 1988 and 1997 [4], the road to Rome. The Rome II criteria for IBS are: abdominal discomfort or pain that has two of three features – relieved with defecation and/or onset associated with a change in frequency of stool and/or onset associated with a change in form of stool are to be present for at least 12 weeks, which need not to be consecutive, in the preceding 12 months (table 3). There are also symptoms cumulatively supporting the diagnosis of IBS: abnormal stool frequency; abnormal stool form; abnormal stool passage; passage of mucus, and bloating or feeling of abdominal distension.

So far two different research approaches have been used to validate gastrointestinal symptoms in IBS. One set of studies has evaluated the discriminatory value of gastrointestinal symptoms in IBS versus health and organic disease. These studies compared gastrointestinal symptoms in patients identified as having IBS with patients who were diagnosed as having organic gastrointestinal disease. In this set no study has attempted to determine if the Rome criteria are of value in discriminating IBS from organic disease [25]. Most of them used gastrointestinal symptoms described by either Manning et al. [26] or Kruis et al. [27] on which the Rome criteria are based.

Table 3. Rome II diagnostic criteria for irritable bowel syndrome

At least 12 weeks, which need not be consecutive, within the preceding 12 months of abdominal discomfort or pain that has two of the following three features	
1	Relieved with defecation
2	Onset associated with a change in frequency of stool
3	Onset associated with a change in form (appearance) of stool

Indeed, the literature on the discriminatory value of gastrointestinal symptoms in organic disease is very limited. Another set of studies has attempted to establish whether gastrointestinal symptoms constitute a true 'syndrome of IBS'. In these, factor analysis has been applied as a statistical method to determine whether there are symptoms that distinctly group together in the population and are consistent with the Rome criteria. It is clear from the available data that although an IBS factor has usually been demonstrated, the symptom items that load on this factor have not generally been consistent. However, only a few of these studies are true population-based studies. Furthermore only some used comprehensive or validated symptom measures limiting the interpretation of the data [25].

Indeed better knowledge of IBS could lead to avoid testing (in particular endoscopy) and thereby saving money. It was estimated that the excess medical cost for diagnosing IBS in the Unites States in 1992 was USD 8 billion [28]. In a recent analysis it has been shown that flexible sigmoidoscopy or colonoscopy constitutes the most costly portion of any work-up for IBS, which amounts to 50–75% of the overall costs [29]. Thus because of their increasingly high cost-effectiveness ratio, endoscopic procedures should not be used at the beginning of the diagnostic work-up but only when a serious organic disease is reasonably likely and needs to be ruled out.

However, there are some controversies regarding these IBS criteria. The change to requiring abdominal pain be present remains controversial. Whether IBS can exist in the absence of abdominal pain is still not settled. It is also not known if these criteria have the same diagnostic value in men as in women. In one study the diagnostic value of the Manning criteria was shown to be of no value in men [30], and women were twice as likely to fulfil the Rome [31] or Manning criteria [32] in random population samples.

These criteria are also quite complex. In a recent report of a population-based study the diagnostic agreement for IBS defined according to the Manning criteria, the Rome II criteria and a simple (Swedish) definition was analysed [30]. The overall agreement of the Swedish definition for IBS compared with the Rome II criteria was 96% whilst compared to Manning criteria it was 90%. The overall agreement between the Manning criteria and the Rome II criteria was 94%. Thus it may be possible to simplify the definition of IBS for epidemiologic studies and clinical practice.

Limits of the Rome Criteria

These criteria are symptom-based and although they were developed by consensus, we still do not have any external diagnostic gold standard. Expert physicians have different training and experience with inevitable personal biases. Symptoms alone are not specific enough for diagnosis and in clinical practice it is mandatory to rule out organic diseases. Thus it is still unknown if these criteria are really able to reduce the number of unnecessary tests increasing the satisfaction of physicians and patients and reducing the costs. Finally there is the risk that the acceptance of these criteria in research and clinical practice might become a self-fulfilling prophecy so that as new scientific data emerge, the capacity to change them may be impaired [34]. Nevertheless the Rome II criteria have standardised the field and promoted clinical research. Their development has been welcomed by regulatory agencies and the pharmaceutical industry despite the criticisms that have arisen. All diagnostic criteria will be controversial until the pathophysiology of IBS is better understood and treatment is more targeted.

References

1 Drossman DA: Psychological and psychophysiologic mechanisms in GI illness; in Kirsner JB (ed): The Growth of Gastroenterologic Knowledge in the 20th Century, ed 1. Philadelphia, Lea & Febiger 1993, pp 419–432.
2 Powell R: On certain painful afflictions of the intestinal canal. Med Trans R Coll Phys 1818; 6:106–117.
3 Cumming W: Electro-galvanism in a peculiar affliction of the mucous membrane of the bowels. Lond Med Gazette 1849;NS9:969–973.
4 Thompson WG: The road to Rome. Gut 1999; 45(suppl 2):II80.
5 Kroenke K, Mangelsdorff AD: Common symptoms in ambulatory care: Incidence, evaluation, therapy, and outcome. Am J Med 1989; 86:262–266.
6 Christensen J: Heraclites or the physician. Gastroenterol Int 1990;3:45–48.
7 Engel GL: The need for a new medical model: A challenge for biomedicine. Science 1977;96: 129–136.
8 Drossman DA: Presidential address: Gastrointestinal illness and biopsychosocial model. Psychosom Med 1998;60:258–267.
9 Thompson WG: The Irritable Bowel Gut. Baltimore, University Park Press, 1979.
10 Drossman DA, Richter JE, Talley NJ: The Functional Gastrointestinal Disorders: Diagnosis, Pathophysiology and Treatment, ed 1. McLean, Degnon, 1994.
11 Drossman DA: The functional gastrointestinal disorders and the Rome II process. Gut 1999; 45(suppl 2):II1–II5.
12 Drossman DA: Do the Rome criteria stand up? in Gobell H, Holtmann G, Talley NJ (eds): Functional Dyspepsia and Irritable Bowel Syndrome: Concepts and Controversies. Falk Symposium 99, ed 1. Dordrecht, Kluwer Academic, 1998, pp 11–18.
13 Whitehead WE: Functional bowel disorders: Are they independent diagnoses? in Corazziari E (ed): Neurogastroentrology, ed 1. Berlin, Gruyter, 1996, pp 65–74.
14 American Psychiatric Association: Diagnostic and Statistical Manual of Mental Disorders-DSM-IV, ed 4. Washington, American Psychiatric Association, 1994.
15 Schumaker HR, Klippel JH, Robinson DR: Primer on the Rheumatic Diseases, ed 9. Atlanta, Arthritis Foundation, 1988.
16 Bayless TM: Inflammatory bowel disease and irritable bowel syndrome. Med Clin North Am 1990;49:21–28.
17 Russo MW, Gaynes BN, Drossman DA: A national survey of practice patterns of gastroenterologists with comparison to the past two decades. J Clin Gastroenterol 1999;29:339–343.
18 Clouse RE, Richter JE, Heading RC, Janssens J, Wilson JA: Functional esophageal disorders. Gut 1999;45(suppl 2):II31–II36.
19 Talley NJ, Stanghellini V, Heading RC, Koch KL, Malegelada JR, Tytgat GNJ: Functional gastrointestinal disorders. Gut 1999;45(suppl 2):II37–II42.
20 Holtmann G, Stanghellini V, Talley NJ: Nomenclature of dyspepsia subgroups and functional dyspepsia: Clarifying the concepts. Baillières Clin Gastroenterol 1998;12:417–433.
21 Stanghellini V: Review article: Pain versus discomfort – Is differentiation clinically useful? Aliment Pharmacol Ther 2001;15:145–149.
22 Carlsson R, Dent J, Bolling-Sternevald E, et al: The usefulness of a structured questionnaire in the assessment of symptomatic gastroesophageal reflux disease. Scand J Gastroenterol 1998;33:1023–1029.
23 Stanghellini V, Tosetti C, Paternico A, De Giorgio R, Barbara G, Salvioli B, Corinaldesi R: Predominant symptoms identify different subgroups in functional dyspepsia. Am J Gastroenterol 1999;94:2080–2085.
24 Talley NJ, Meineche-Schmidt V, Pare P, et al: Efficacy of omeprazole in functional dyspepsia: Double blind, randomised placebo controlled trials. Aliment Pharmacol Ther 1998;12:1055–1065.

25 Hammer J, Talley NJ: Diagnostic criteria for the irritable bowel syndrome. Am J Med 1999; 107:5S–11S.
26 Manning AP, Thompson WG, Heaton KW, Morris AF: Towards positive diagnosis of the irritable bowel. Br Med J 1978;ii:653–654.
27 Kruis W, Thieme C, Weinzierl M, Schussier P, Holl J, Paulus W: A diagnostic score for the irritable bowel syndrome: Its value in the exclusion of organic disease. Gastroenterology 1984; 87:1–7.
28 Talley NJ, Gabriel SE, Harmsen WS, Zinsmeister AR, Evans RW: Medical costs in community subjects with irritable bowel syndrome. Gastroenterology 1995;109:1736–1741.
29 Suleiman S, Sonnenberg A: Cost-effectiveness of endoscopy in irritable bowel syndrome. Arch Intern Med 2001;161:369–375.
30 Smith RC, Greenbaum DS, Vancouver JB, et al: Gender differences in Manning criteria in the irritable bowel syndrome. Gastroenterology 1991;101:591–595.
31 Drossman DA, Li Z, Andruzzi E, et al: US householder survey of functional gastrointestinal disorders: Prevalence, sociodemography and health impact. Dig Dis Sci 1993;38:1569–1580.
32 Heaton KW, O'Donnel LJD, Braddon FEM, Mountford RA, Hughes AO, Cripps PJ: Symptoms of irritable bowel syndrome in a British urban community: Consulters and non-consulters. Gastroenterology 1992;102:1962–1967.
33 Agreus L, Talley NJ, Svardsudd K, Tibblin G, Jones MP: Identifying dyspepsia and irritable bowel syndrome: The value of pain or discomfort, and bowel habit descriptors. Scand J Gastroenterol 2000;35:142–151.
34 Drossman DA: The Rome criteria process: Diagnosis and legitimization of irritable bowel syndrome. Am J Gastroenterol 1999;94:2803–2807.

Review Article

Digestive Diseases

Dig Dis 2001;19:232–239

Tests for the Evaluation of Functional Gastrointestinal Disorders

C. Knippig[a] R. Fass[b] P. Malfertheiner[a]

[a]Department of Gastroenterology, University of Magdeburg, Germany;
[b]GI Motility Laboratories, University of Arizona, Tucson, Ariz., USA

Key Words

Function tests, esophageal, gastric, intestinal · Manometry · Barostat · Functional imaging

Abstract

Functional gastrointestinal disorders are a common problem. Different noninvasive and invasive strategies have been carried out in recent years to study the role of impaired myoelectrical activity, tone, compliance, transit and perception of the gastrointestinal tract. Esophageal barostat examination and impedance measurements have been added to standard clinical methods like manometry and pH-metry for the esophagus. Bilirubin measurement allows the evaluation of duodenogastroesophageal reflux and perception can be studied by gastric barostat. Electrogastrography and tenostat test are still research tools. Rectal or sigmoid barostat examination is a new research tool to study visceral sensitivity in the lower gastrointestinal tract. New methods – like functional MRI and SPECT – are promising features for the future.

'To eat is human, digest divine'
Mark Twain

Physicians that are asked to evaluate abdominal symptoms are often left with no answer, even after a battery of imaging studies have been ordered. Consequently, a diagnosis of exclusion is made – functional disorder (table 1). To further investigate the impaired function or abnormal perception of the gastrointestinal tract, a wide variety of tests and research tools have become available. Alterations in perception and motility may lead to discomfort, bloating or pain. Evaluation of functional disorders include invasive or noninvasive tests that allow us to examine various pathophysiological aspects of functional disorders of the gastrointestinal tract, which include myoelectrical activity, tone, compliance, transit and perception. The aim of this article is to provide an up-to-date review of the different techniques to study gastrointestinal function for clinical and research purposes.

Esophagus

Typical esophageal symptoms include heartburn, acid regurgitation and dysphagia. Rumination syndrome and globus sensation are less common. In patients with esophageal related symptoms and a negative endoscopy, functional tests that include esophageal manometry and 24-

KARGER

Fax + 41 61 306 12 34
E-Mail karger@karger.ch
www.karger.com

0257–2753/01/0193–0232$17.50/0

Accessible online at:
www.karger.com/journals/ddi

Prof. Dr. med. P. Malfertheiner
Department of Gastroenterology, Otto-von-Guericke University of Magdeburg
Leipziger Strasse 44, D–39120 Magdeburg (Germany)
Tel. +49 391 671 31 50, Fax +49 391 671 31 05
E-Mail peter.malfertheiner@medizin.uni-magdeburg.de

hour esophageal pH monitoring are ordered based on patients' symptoms. Esophageal barostat may be added to diagnose esophageal hypersensitivity. Adequate explanation about the techniques and their risks is needed prior to every diagnostic test.

Esophageal Manometry

Esophageal manometry is the gold standard to detect motility disorders of the esophagus. Evaluation of the amplitude of the esophageal contraction wave, its configuration and propagation as well as the function of the upper and lower esophageal sphincters (LES) may be provided. The first measurements were carried out by Arloing and Kronecker more than 100 years ago. A continuously water-perfused manometry system was introduced in the 1960s [1]. The solid-state manometry system allowed ambulatory esophageal motility recordings. Today both systems are in use, however, the water-perfused stationary manometry system is the most common. The stationary water-perfused esophageal manometry provides reliable assessment of the lower esophageal sphincter function via a sleeve catheter and can diagnose most motility disorders, such as achalasia and diffuse esophageal spasm. In patients with retrosternal chest pain and normal stationary esophageal manometry, one should consider performing 24-hour esophageal manometry. The new topographical method uses 21 intraluminal recording sites instead of the regular 4, may be more accurate in diagnosing the type of esophageal motor dysfunction and provide additional information that is important in the clinical practice of esophageal manometry [2]. Furthermore, it is possible to detect incomplete LES relaxations in patients with normal results with the standard methods. Additionally, improvement in the identification of the upper margin of the lower sphincter has been reported. In recent years a miniature esophageal manometric technique has been developed and appears to provide very good clinical data [3].

Clinical value: Esophageal manometry is a commonly used standard procedure in clinical practice. Indications for the procedure are given in table 2. In acid reflux disease the resting LES pressure and length, as well as motility disorder of the esophageal body, are considered the most important preoperative parameters. However, different esophageal motility abnormalities can be seen in the esophageal body of patients with acid reflux disease. Improvement after Nissen-Rossetti fundoplication suggests that these disorders may be a secondary motor dysfunction. However, there is a lack of complete normalization in motor activity postoperatively indicating an additional partially primary impairment of motor activity [4].

Table 1. Functional esophageal disorders

Primary motility disorders
Nutcracker esophagus
Diffuse esophageal spasm
Achalasia/Chagas' disease
Disorders of LES function
Ineffective peristalsis
Secondary motility disorders
Systemic sclerosis, CREST
Iatrogenic: surgical, medications
Diabetes mellitus

Table 2. Indications for esophageal manometry [1]

Dysphagia
Noncardiac chest pain
Systemic diseases (e.g. scleroderma, connective tissue disorders)
Before antireflux surgery
Achalasia

In noncardiac chest pain esophageal manometry should be considered if pH testing is unremarkable as spastic motility disorders may be the reason for patients' symptoms. pH-metry should be used initially, preferably after treatment failure [7]. Esophageal barostat may have a role in determining those patients with symptoms due to visceral hyperalgesia. However, it has to be considered that cardiac manipulation itself can induce esophageal motility abnormalities and coronary angioplasty is associated with esophageal hyperalgesia – the cardio-esophageal reflex – suggesting that patients' symptoms can be the result of triggering both diseases.

Manometric variations in achalasia have been divided into four subcategories: (a) the presence of high amplitude esophageal body contractions; (b) a short segment of esophageal body aperistalsis; (c) retained complete deglutitive LES relaxation, and (d) intact transient LES relaxation [8]. Complete LES relaxation that was observed in some achalasia patients appears to be functionally inadequate (abnormally short duration) [9]. In the late phase of the disease, nonperistaltic, low-amplitude contractions appear and represent a 'common cavity' phenomenon. This is due to dilatation of the esophageal corpus, which does not allow any detection of contractions with the manometric catheter. Using special catheters, a manometrically guided endoscopic injection of botulinum toxin is possible and is associated with increased safety and efficacy of therapy [10].

In contrast to motility disorders of the esophageal corpus or LES, impaired function of the upper esophageal sphincter should be evaluated by an additional radiologic method – like videocine esophagram – as manometry itself may not be sufficiently sensitive [11–13]. However, in specific diseases like Kearns-Syre syndrome and chronic progressive external ophthalmoplegia [14], cricopharyngeal achalasia can be detected by upper esophageal manometry [14].

Table 3. Gastric and small bowel functional disorders

Primary functional disorders	
	Dyspepsia
	Chronic intestinal pseudo-obstruction
	Sphincter of Oddi dysfunction
Secondary motility disorders	
	Diabetes mellitus
	Iatrogenic: surgical, medications
	Myopathies, neuropathies

pH-Metry, Bilirubin and Impedance Evaluation

Ambulatory 24-hour pH-metry is indicated in patients who failed standard dose PPI, candidates for antireflux surgery and possibly in patients with extraesophageal manifestations of GERD. However, pH-metry is not a valid method for the measurement of duodenogastroesophageal reflux. Monitoring of bilirubin is possible via a fiberoptic bilirubin catheter (Bilitec, Synetics Medical, Sweden). An additional new diagnostic tool for detection of nonacid reflux is the impedance planimetry method.

Clinical value: In patients with extraesophageal manifestations of GERD, the pH catheter is positioned as previously described with the second sensor 5 cm below the UES. However, we and others found no additional diagnostic value for the second pH sensor.

Bilirubin examinations should only be performed in specialized centers as clinical value for routine usage seems to be very low [15]. Isolated esophageal bilirubin reflux in patients with an intact stomach is uncommon [15]. However, some studies found a significant difference in bilirubin exposure between long-segment Barrett's esophagus and GERD, whereas there was no significant difference between short-segment Barrett's esophagus compared to GERD, hinting to different etiopathology of both long- and short-segment Barrett's esophagus [16]. However, it has to be emphasized that bilirubin is only a pigment and the actual method is lacking the capability of detecting bile salts, which play an important role in the pathophysiology of mucosal injury and patients' symptoms. Using impedance method it has been demonstrated that one third of reflux events is nonacid in GERD [17], however, the clinical value of this finding is still under evaluation.

Esophageal Barostat

Barostat, a computerized distension device, allows examination of visceral sensitivity by controlled balloon inflations in the desired organ – esophagus, stomach or sigmoid/rectum. The barostat system includes a small polyethylene balloon that is connected via a cannula to a volume- or pressure-controlled hydraulic pump.

Clinical value: The tool is still experimental and its specific role in clinical practice has yet to be determined. However, it has been suggested to be useful in evaluating patients with non-GERD-related NCCP and functional heartburn [18–20].

Gastric and Small Intestinal Functional Testing

Typical gastric symptomatology includes epigastric pain, discomfort, a 'knot-like' feeling in the stomach, early satiety, nausea and vomiting. These symptoms can be related to different primary or secondary functional disorders (table 3). The most common gastric functional testing is the examination of gastric emptying, followed by antroduodenal manometry and gastric barostat.

Evaluation of Gastric Emptying

History: Gastric emptying measurements have switched from expensive and invasive methods to less expensive, noninvasive tests like ^{13}C-octaonic or -acetate breath tests. Scintigraphic methods have been commonly used for gastric emptying assessment in the last decade. These methods are easy to perform, noninvasive and allow additional evaluation of antral contraction patterns and intragastric meal distribution [21]. However, rising costs, the need for radiation and interindividual difficulties in the definition of area of interest have forced the evaluation of new strategies. Although scintigraphic methods are still in use, a modification that uses less time points (1, 2 and 4 h after meals) has recently been validated and shown to bo cost-effective in a recent multinational study [22].

The radiopaque marker is a simple and readily available method that can be used where no other methods are available. This modality has been compared to scintigraphy and was found to be equally reliable [23]. The need for radiologic exponation of patients as well as the inability to achieve more detailed analyses of gastric emptying led to the development of various technologies. Ultrasonographic evaluation of gastric emptying was first described by Stein et al. [24] in 1972 followed by Bateman and Whittingham [25]. The method was modified to sagittal antrum planimetry and validated against scintigraphic procedures [26]. However, gastric ultrasonographic examination is time-consuming and can only be used with liquid meals. Due to artifacts, a solid meal does not allow correct measurements in the distal antral wall. Other methods like the metal detector [27] or impedance [28] were not found to have a clinical role.

Stable nonradioactive isotope methods, ^{13}C bound either to acetate or octaonic acid, are currently replacing scintigraphic methods. ^{13}C can be labeled to the solid phase of a meal, e.g. egg. When the substrate is absorbed it is metabolized in the liver and then excreted into the blood from where $^{13}CO_2$ is transported to the lung and then can be monitored in patients' breath. Breath tests are easy to perform and have been validated against scintigraphy. No radiologic exponation like in the radiopaque marker method, or invasive strategies, like the former intubation methods, have to be used. The breath test has been shown to be useful in clinical and research analyses. Functional MRI measurement is a new technique that includes three-dimensional evaluation of gastric emptying and leads to a complete new view of the pathophysiology of gastric emptying (see below) [29–39].

Clinical value: Evaluation of gastric emptying is a routine procedure. The most common indication is the evaluation of gastric emptying in patients with diabetes mellitus [40, 41]. However, hyperglycemia has been shown to delay gastric emptying, and hypoglycemia to accelerate gastric emptying. Therefore, evaluation of gastric emptying in diabetes only makes sense in patients with good glucose control.

Electrogastrography (EGG)

EGG is a new diagnostic tool which was primarily invented to study gastric myoelectric activity. Nowadays, EGG measurements allow to distinguish distinct patient subgroups [42]. However, the clinical utility of EGG is still being evaluated. EGG was first performed in 1921 by Alvarez and colleagues. Presently, different EGG electrodes are used. Two electrodes are usually placed on the abdomen after 8 h of fasting. Detection of gastric myeloelectric activity is possible with the help of either a portable recorder or a stationary unit at a frequency of at least 4 Hz. Simultaneous measurement of gastric emptying or antroduodenal motility is recommended.

Clinical value: Primarily, patients with impaired gastric emptying and suspected antral motor dysfunction are studied [42]. However, most electrogastrographic patterns are nonspecific [43]. Thus, it has been mainly used to detect dysrhythmia in patients with diabetes or functional dyspepsia.

Gastric Barostat

Controlled inflation of an intragastric polyethylene balloon is a very intriguing method to evaluate reflex motor function of the fundus. Perception thresholds during balloon distension as well as drug [44, 45] or meal-induced fundus relaxation can be studied.

Clinical value: Different diseases have been shown to result in impaired fundic accommodation and gastric perception. Gastric hypersensitivity [46] and an impaired fundic accommodation [47] may play an important role in functional dyspepsia. However, in functional dyspepsia, individual symptoms are not a predictor for the presence of gastric hypersensitivity [48]. Additionally, impaired postprandial gastric relaxation has also been demonstrated in GERD, diabetes mellitus, acute hyper- or hypoglycemia and achalasia [5, 49–53]. The test is invasive, time-consuming and may produce discomfort in patients and potentially vagal dysregulation. Technically, the effect of the balloon itself and the possible induction of 'iatrogenic' disorders [54] have to be evaluated in further studies.

Tenostat Test

Gastric wall tension is a factor that can be assessed by the new tenostat test in addition to the conventional gastric barostat. The tenostat consists of a controlled air pump combined with a strain gauge independently connected via a double-lumen polyvinyl tube to an intragastric bag. According to Laplace's law (Tension = pressure × radius/2), tension is then calculated (g/cm).

Clinical value: The tenostat test is a research tool. Although there are still some methodological problems to be resolved, there is already some evidence that perception of gastric distension depends on wall tension rather than on intraluminal pressure or volume [42].

Functional Ultrasound

Ultrasound examination is a noninvasive, easy to perform and widely available method that can lead to valid and reproducible functional data. It has been used to assess gallbladder emptying and contractility as well as to assess the effect of meals on bile duct diameter.

Clinical value: The esophageal junction can best be visualized in children up to 5 years of age with a 100% sensitivity and 87.5% specificity as compared to ambulatory pH testing for diagnosis of GERD. Gallbladder ultrasound is also a valid method with clinical benefit in dysmotility-like dyspepsia, gallstone disease and drug efficacy. Common bile duct measurements, inter- and postprandially, are done in patients with clinical suspicion of common bile duct obstruction [55].

Antroduodenal/Antrojejunal Manometry

To study antroduodenal/antrojejunal motility patterns – fasting and postprandially – manometry is considered to be the gold standard. The procedure is indicated in subgroups of patients with unexplained upper gastrointestinal symptoms, primarily when pseudo-obstruction is suspected.

Clinical value: Antroduodenal/antrojejunal manometry is not routinely performed. However, it is a useful tool to study the pathophysiology of special diseases. Differentiation between neuronal or muscular disorders that affect the stomach and proximal small bowel is possible [42]. However, it is a time-consuming diagnostic tool and there is still the question of whether the motility disorders documented are related to the patients' symptoms [56]. New insights into circadian variation in antroduodenal motor activity and improved patients' acceptance may be the consequence of new portable recording systems [57, 58].

Abnormalities of gastropyloroduodenal motility have been shown in functional dyspepsia during interdigestive and digestive stages, which included a higher incidence of isolated pyloric pressure waves [59]. However, the main indication for antroduodenal manometry remains the suspicion of pseudo-obstruction [60]. Antroduodenal characteristics of the latter include short or prolonged bursts of nonpropagating activity in the fasting and/or fed state [61]. Additional studies have been performed in achalasia [62], hyperglycemia and hyperinsulinemia [63] as well as in diabetes mellitus [64]. Documented abnormalities may be useful in explaining patients' symptoms and delayed gastric emptying.

Colonic and Anorectal Functional Disorders

Lower gastrointestinal symptoms include mainly bloating, abdominal discomfort, constipation and diarrhea. Functional diseases of the lower gastrointestinal tract can be grouped into primary and secondary disorders (table 4). Functional evaluation is primarily done by determining of transit time as well as colonic or anorectal motility via manometry. Perception thresholds can be measured by rectal or sigmoid distensions.

Table 4. Colonic and anorectal functional disorders

Primary functional disorders
Irritable bowel syndrome
Constipation
Fecal incontinence
Secondary functional disorders
Iatrogenic intervention
Medication
Surgery

Transit Time

Transit abnormalities of the upper gastrointestinal tract and colon are common in patients with functional related gastrointestinal symptoms. Patients with constipation tend to predominately have delayed colonic transit. Transit disorders can be evaluated with the help of the radiopaque marker method (Sitz Mark Study [40]). However, a more sophisticated method, a scintigraphic evaluation that uses ^{99m}Tc and ^{111}In DTPA, can be performed to evaluate a whole gut transit [65]. Both methods allow determination of the section of the digestive tract that is responsible for abnormal gut motility. New methods, like MRI measurements, are under evaluation.

Clinical value: Scintigraphic methods and the radiopaque marker method are both simple and clinically useful tests. However, scintigraphic evaluation is more expensive but allows a more sophisticated evaluation of gastrointestinal motility.

Rectal Manometry

Rectal manometry was introduced in the 1930s with the help of the balloon catheter [1]. Nowadays, the combined water perfusion catheter system with a balloon at its tip is the commonly used assembly which causes less irritation.

Clinical value: Anorectal manometry is clinically indicated in patients with suspected fecal incontinence. More sophisticated analyses of structural abnormalities postpartum or surgery are possible via vector analyses. Colonic manometry is a modality that is available only in

Table 5. Functional testing of the gastrointestinal tract

Primarily for routine use	Primarily for clinical research
Esophageal and anorectal manometry	Bilirubin and impedance planimetry
pH testing	Esophageal, gastric and rectal barostat
(Antroduodenal manometry)	Tenostat
Gastric emptying evaluation	EGG
(scintigraphy or breath test)	Functional ultrasound
Radiographic marker studies	Colonic manometry
	Antroduodenal/antrojejunal manometry
	FMRI, SPECT

specialized centers as a research tool. In children with chronic intestinal pseudo-obstruction, a high frequency of constipation can be seen. In the colon of patients with pseudo-obstruction, an absence of high amplitude propagating contractions and gastrocolonic response or complete disappearance of colonic contractions has been demonstrated [66].

Rectal Barostat
Rectal barostat examination is performed in patients with clinically suspected irritable bowel syndrome. Visceral hypersensitivity appears to play a major pathogenetic role in these patients [67].

Clinical value: In patients with irritable bowel syndrome a reduction of perception thresholds for pain can be observed (compared to healthy controls) as evidence of visceral hypersensitivity [68, 69, 74]. However, rectal barostat is not a tool for routine clinical assessment and is currently used solely for research purposes. Additionally, some patients with diagnosis of irritable bowel syndrome may not demonstrate visceral hypersensitivity. Rectal distension is used in pathophysiological studies of the brain-gut axis by simultaneous evaluation of cerebral activation by magnetic resonance imaging (MRI).

fMRI (Functional Magnetic Resonance Imaging) and SPECT (Single Photon Emission Computed Tomography) – The Future?

As has been suggested for a long period of time, some symptoms 'are in the patient's head'. PET and fMRI have been recently used for functional evaluation of the gastrointestinal tract. Whereas the first functional MRI studies focused on the gastrointestinal tract per se – like gastric emptying and gastric accommodation [37, 70] – current studies concentrate on the brain-gut interaction aspect by measuring cerebral activation in response to intraluminal stimuli.

Gastric emptying is best evaluated by adding gadolinium-acetic acid to a standardized liquid meal. T1-weighted scans are performed in predetermined time intervals in the supine position. Gastric emptying, contractions and secretion can be evaluated. Three-dimensional views are obtainable. A correlation to scintigraphic study of gastric emptying has been shown. In some specialized units, patients are examined by cerebral fMRI for regional brain activation by setting gastrointestinal stimuli. An example is the usage of balloon distensions delivered by a barostat. This requires a special MRI technique (fast acquisition rate) and software.

For SPECT evaluation, ^{99m}Tc-pertechnate is taken up by the gastric mucosa. Tomographic images of the stomach are acquired by a dual-headed gamma camera system. In combination with transaxial images, three-dimensional images can be reconstructed and total gastric volume as well as secretion can be assessed at baseline and postprandially [42].

Clinical use: fMRI and SPECT are mainly used to study physiology, pathophysiology and drug effect on the gastrointestinal tract. New studies are concentrating on the effect of gastrointestinal stimulation, like distension on cerebral activation. The actual fMRI method is time-consuming and expensive to be used in clinical practice [71, 72]. However, by reducing measurements to special time points postprandially, the cost could be further reduced and the clinical utility increased.

There are still some technical problems to be resolved. High interobserver variability in SPECT evaluation (12–13%) that requires modifications. However, the intraobserver variance coefficients of 8–9% are promising. Gastric barostat or the water/nutrient test should be added, as symptoms of patients are not assessed in the actual protocols [73].

Conclusion

Diagnostic methods for functional gastrointestinal diseases are major tools for future research. Besides the standard clinical evaluation the new diagnostic tools offer large amounts of information. This includes the barostat and the usage of MRI and SPECT (table 5). However, technical problems and cost need to be addressed in the future before these methods become useful in everyday clinical practice.

References

1 Karaus M, Allescher HD: Manometrie von Ösophagus und Anorektum. Leitlinien des Arbeitskreises Gastrointestinale Motilität und Funktion eV (under review).

2 Cluse RE, Staiano A, Alrakawi A, Haroian L: Application of topographical methods to clinical esophageal manometry. Am J Gastroenterol 2000,95:2677–2678.

3 Shanmuganathan G, Ritz MA, Holloway RH, Di Matteo AC, Omari TI: Evaluation of miniature manometric techniques for the measurement of esophageal body pressure waves. J Gastroenterol Hepatol 2000;15:1362–1369.

4 Wallner G, Zgodzinski W, Skoczylas T, Misiuna P: Esophageal motility impairment – the cause or consequence of gastroesophageal reflux disease. Przegl Lek 2000;57(suppl 5):89–91.

5 Undeland KA, Hausken T, Aanderud S, Berstad A: Lower postprandial gastric volume response in diabetic patients with vagal neuropathy. Neurogastroenterol Motil 1997;9:19–24.

6 Boulant J, Mathieu S, Dàmato M, Abergel A, Dapoigny M, Bommelaer G: Cholecystokinin in transient lower oesophageal sphincter relaxation due to gastric distension in humans. Gut 1997;40:57–81.

7 Shrestha S, Pasricha PJ: Update on noncardiac chest pain. Dig Dis 2000;18:138–146.

8 Hirano I, Tatum RP, Shi G, Sang Q, Joehl RJ, Kahrilas P: Manometric heterogeneity in patients with idiopathic achalasia. Gastroenterology 2001;120:789–798.

9 Mearin F, Malagelada JR: Complete lower esophageal sphincter relaxation observed in some achalasia patients is functionally inadequate. Am J Physiol 2000;278:G376–G383.

10 Wehrmann T, Schmitt T, Dietrich CF, Caspary WF, Seifert H: Manometrically-guided endoscopic injection of botulinum toxin for esophageal achalasia: A pilot trial. Z Gastroenterol 2000;38:899–903.

11 Motil KJ, Schultz RJ, Browning K, Trautwein L, Glaze DG: Oropharyngeal dysfunction and gastroesophageal dysmotility are present in girls and women with Rett syndrome. J Pediatr Gastroenterol Nutr 1999;29:31–37.

12 Dantas RO: Upper esophageal sphincter pressure in patients with Chagas' disease and primary achalasia. Braz J Med Biol Res 2000;33:545–551.

13 Malhi-Chowla N, Achem SR, Stark ME, DeVault KR: Manometry of the upper esophageal sphincter and pharynx is not useful in unselected patients referred for esophageal testing. Am J Gastroenterol 2000;95:1417–1421.

14 Kornblum C, Broicher R, Walther E, Seibel P, Reichmann H, Klockgether T, Herberhold C, Schröder R: Cricopharyngeal achalasia is a common cause of dysphagia in patients with mtDNA deletions. Neurology 2001;56:1409–1412.

15 Marshall RE, Anggiansah A, Owen WA, Owen WJ: Investigation of gastro-oesophaeal reflux in patients with an intact stomach: Is oesophageal bilirubin monitoring a useful addition to pH monitoring? Scand J Gastroenterol 2000;35:904–909.

16 Pfaffenbach B, Hullerum J, Orth KH, Langer M, Stabenow-Lohbauer U, Lux G: Bile and acid reflux in long and short segment Barretts esophagus, and in reflux disease. Z Gastroenterol 2000;38:565–570.

17 Sifrim D, Holloway R, Silny J, Xin Z, Tack J, Lerut A, Janssens J: Acid, nonacid, and gas reflux in patients with gastroesophageal reflux disease during ambulatory 24-hour pH-impedance recordings. Gastroenterology 2001;120:1588–1598.

18 Hu WH, Marin CJ, Talley NJ: Intraesophageal acid perfusion sensitizes the esophagus to mechanical distension: A barostat study. Am J Gastroenterol 2000;95:2189–2194.

19 Shi G, Tatum RP, Joehl RJ, Kahriilas PJ: Esophageal sensitivity and symptom perception in gastroesophaeal reflux disease. Curr Gastroenterol Rep 1999;1:214–219.

20 Mujica VR, Mudipalli RS, Rao SS: Pathophysiology of chest pain in patients with nutcracker esophagus. Am J Gastroenterol 2001;96:1371–1377.

21 Fried M: Methods to study gastric emptying: Moderator's comments. Dig Dis Sci 1994;39:114S–115S.

22 Tougas G, Chen Y, Coates G: Standardization of a simplified scintigraphic methodology for the assessment of gastric emptying in a multicenter setting. Am J Gastroenterology 2000;95:78–86.

23 Stotzer PO, Fjalling M, Gretarsdottir J, Abrahamsson H: Assessment of gastric emptying: Comparison of solid scintigraphic emptying and emptying of radiopaque markers in patients and healthy subjects. Dig Dis Sci 1999;44:729–734.

24 Stein WW, Brettel HF, Garten Th: Volumenbestimmung des Mageninhaltes mit dem Ultraschall-B-Bildverfahren. MMW 1972;114:1871–1873.

25 Bateman DN, Whittingham TA: Gastric emptying measurement by real-time ultrasound. Z Gastroenterol 1981;19:417.

26 Tympner F, Feldmeier J, Rösch W: Korrelationsstudie der sonographischen mit den szintigraphischen Messergebnissen der Magenentleerung. Ultraschall Med 1986;7:264–267.

27 Eberschaer B, Ewe K, Alles U, Schmidtmann I: Effect of 4 × 250 mg erythromycin on human gastrointestinal transit. Z Gastroenterol 1995;33:340–344.

28 Sutton JA, Thompson S, Sobnack R: Measurement of gastric emptying rates by radioactive isotope scanning and epigastric impedance. Lancet 1985;i:898–900.

29 Gerards C, Tromm A: Verfahren zur Messung der Magenentleerung. Leber Magen Darm 1999;29:128–138.

30 Bateman DN, Whittingham TA: Gastric emptying measurement by real-time ultrasound. Z Gastroenterol 1981;19:417.

31 Beaumont W: Experiments and observations on the gastric juice and the physiology of digestion. Plattsburgh, Allen, 1833.

32 Braaden B, Adams S, Duan LP, Orth KH, Maul FD, Lembcke B, Hör, G, Caspary F: The ^{13}C-acetate breath test accurately reflects gastric emptying of liquids in both liquid and semisolid test meals. Gastroenterology 1995;108:1048–1055.

33 Chaudhuri TK: Use of ^{99m}Tc-DTPA for measuring gastric emptying time. J Nucl Med 1974;15:391–395.

34 Chen J, McCallum RW: Clinical application of electrogastrography. Am J Gastroenterol 1993;88:1324–1336.

35 Chitsakul K, Bouchoucha M, Lee JW, Cugnenc PH: A new system for gastric emptying analysis using impedance measurement. Arch Int Physiol Biochem Biophys 1994;102:71–76.

36 Ewe K, Press AG, Dederer W: Gastrointestinal transit of indigestible solids measured by metal detector EAS II. Eur J Clin Invest 1989;19:291–297.

37 Fraser R, Schwizer W, Boroviicka J, Asal K, Fried M: Gastric motility measurement by MRI. Dig Dis Sci 1994;39:S20–S23.

38 Gerards C, Tromm A, May B: Optimierung der sonographischen Antrumplanimetrie zur sonographischen Bestimmung der Magenentleerung mit Hilfe der Entleerungsfunktionsgeraden. Ultraschall Med 1998;19:83–86.
39 Ghoos YFG, Maes BD, Geypens BJ, Mys G, Hiele MI, Rutgeerts PJ, Vantrappen G: Measurement of gastric emptying rate of solids by means of a carbon-labeled octaonic acid breath test. Gastroenterology 1993;104:1640–1647.
40 Iida M, Ikeda M, Kishimoto M, Tsujino T, Kaneto H, Matsuhisa M, Kajimoto Y, Watarai T, Ymasaki Y, Hori M: Evaluation of gut motility in type II diabetes by the radiopaque marker method. J Gastroenterol Hepatol 2000; 15:381–385.
41 Kong MF, Horowitz M: Gastric emptying in diabetes mellitus: Relationship to blood-glucose control. Clin Geriatr Med 1999;15:321–338.
42 Kim DY, Myung SJ, Camilleri M: Novel testing of human gastric motor and sensory functions: Rationale, methods and potential applications in clinical practice. Am J Gastroenterol 2000;95:3365–3373.
43 Kauer WK, Stein HJ, Balint A, Siewert JR: Transcutaneous electrogastrography: A non-invasive method to evaluate post-operative gastric disorders? Hepatogastroenterology 1999; 46:1244–1248.
44 Levein NG, Thorn SE, Lindberg G, Wattwill M: Dopamine reduces gastric tone in a dose-related manner. Acta Anaesthesiol Scand 1999; 43:722–725.
45 Tack J, Broeckaert D, Coulie B, Janssens J: The influence of cisapride on gastric tone and the perception on gastric distension. Aliment Pharmacol Ther 1998;12:761–766.
46 Rhee PL, Kim YH, Son HJ, Kim JJ, Koh KC, Paik SW, Rhee JC: The etiologic role of gastric hypersensitivity in functional dyspepsia in Korea. J Clin Gastroenterol 1999;29:332–335.
47 Tack J: Functional dyspepsia: Impaired fundic accommodation. Curr Treat Options Gastroenterol 2000;3:287–294.
48 Rhee PL, Kim YH, Son HJ, Kim JJ, Koh KC, Paik SW, Rhee JC, Choi KW: Evaluation of individual symptoms cannot predict presence of hypersensitivity in functional dyspepsia. Dig Dis Sci 2000;45:1680–1684.
49 Zerbib F, des Varannes SB, Ropert A, Lamouliatte H, Quinton A, Galmiche JP: Proximal gastric tone in gastro-oesophageal reflux disease. Eur J Gastroenterol Hepatol 1999;11: 511–515.
50 Van Petersen AS, Vu MK, Lam WF, Lamers CB, Ringers J, Masclee AA: Effects of hyperglycemia and hyperinsulinaemia on proximal motor and sensory function in humans. Clin Sci (Colch) 2000;99:37–46.
51 Verhagen MA, Rayner CK, Andrews JM, Hebbard GS, Doran SM, Horowitz M: Physiological changes in blood glucose do not affect gastric compliance and perception in normal subjects. Am J Physiol 1999;276:G761–G766.
52 Bittinger M, Barnert J, Eberl T, Wienbeck M: Postprandial gastric relaxation in achalasia. Eur J Gastoenterol Hepatol 1998;10:741–744.
53 Samsom M, Roelofs JM, Akkermans LM, van Berge Heegouwen GP: Proximal gastric motor activity in response to a liquid meal in diabetes mellitus with autonomic neuropathy. Dig Dis Sci 1998;43:491–496.
54 Samsom M, Hauskens T, Mundt M: Gastric accommodation is influenced by the presence of an intragastric balloon. Gastroenterology 2000;118:A621.
55 Portincasa P, Colecchia A, Dia Ciaula A, Larocca A, Muraca M, Palasciano G, Roda E, Festi D: Standards for diagnosis of gastrointestinal motility disorders. Section Ultrasonography. A position statement from the Gruppo Italiano di Studio Motilità Apparato Digerente. Dig Liver Dis 2000;32:160–172.
56 Verhagen MA, Samsom M, Jebbink RJ, Smout AJ: Clinical relevance of antroduodenal manometry. Eur J Gastroenterol Hepatol 1999;11: 523–528.
57 Bortolotti M, Annese V, Coccia G: Twenty-four-hour ambulatory antroduodenal manometry in normal subjects (cooperative study). Neurogastroenterol Motil 2000;12:231–238.
58 Penning C, Gielkens HA, Hemelaar M, Delemarre JB, Bemelman WA, Lamers CB, Masclee AA: Prolonged ambulatory recording of antroduodenal motility in slow transit constipation. Br J Surg 2000;87:211–217.
59 Gu C, Ke M, Wang Z: Temporal and spatial relationship of pylorus to antroduodenal motility in functional dyspepsia. Chin Med J (Engl) 1998;111:906–909.
60 Martinez Martinez L, Lopez Santamaria M, Prieto Bozano G, Molina Arias M, Jimenez Alvarez C, Tovar Larrucea JA: Diagnosis and therapeutic options in chronic idiopathic intestinal pseudo-obstruction: Review of 16 cases. Cir Pediatr 1999;12:71–74.
61 Cucchiara S, Borrelli O, Salvia G, Iula VDD, Fecarotta S, Gaudiello G, Boccia G, Annese V: A normal gastrointestinal motility excludes chronic intestinal pseudo-obstruction in children. Dig Dis Sci 2000;45:258–264.
62 Verhagen MA, Samsom M, Smout AJ: Gastric myoelectrical and antroduodenal motor activity in patients with achalasia. Neurogastroenterol Motil 1998;10:211–218.
63 Gielkens HA, Verkijk M, Frolich M, Lamers CB, Masclee AA: Is the effect of acute hyperglycaemia on interdigestive antroduodenal motility and small bowel transit mediated by insulin? Eur J Clin Invest 1997;27:703–710.
64 Samsom M, Jebbink RJ, Akktermans LM, Van Berge-Henegouwens GB, Smout AJ: Abnormalities of antroduodenal motility in type I diabetes. Diabetes Care 1996;19:21–27.
65 Bonapace ES, Maurer AH, Davidoff S, Krevsky Fisher RS, Parkman HP: Whole gut transit scintigraphy in the clinical evaluation of patients with upper and lower gastrointestinal symptoms. Am J Gastroenterol 2000;95:2838–2847.
66 Di Lorenzo C, Flores AF, Reddy SN, Snape WJ Jr, Bazzocchi G, Hyman PE: Colonic manometry in children with chronic intestinal pseudo-obstruction. Gut 1993;34:803–807.
67 Mayer EA, Gebhart GF: Basic and clinical aspects of visceral hyperalgesia. Gastroenterology 1994;107:291–293.
68 Boulant J, Fioramonti J, Dapogny M, Bommelaer G, Bueno L: Cholecystokinin and nitric oxide in transient lower esophageal sphincter relaxation to gastric distension in dogs. Gastroenterology 1994;107:1059–1066.
69 Zigelboim J Talley NJ, Phillips SF: Response of gastric fundus to rectal distension in healthy persons. Dig Dis Sci 1994;39:1441–1445.
70 Choi MG, Kim BW, Choo KY: Measurement of gastric accommodation and emptying of a solid meal by magnetic resonance imaging. Gastroenterology 2000;118:A388–A389.
71 Feinle C, Kunz P, Boesinger P: Scintigraphic validation of a magnetic resonance imaging method to study gastric emptying of a solid meal in humans. Gut 1999;44:106–111.
72 Faas HM, Rades T, Roche HL: Measurement of intragastric distribution of drugs by MRI in humans – a liposomal drug model. Gastroenterology 1999;116:A991.
73 Kuiken SD, Samson M, Camilleri M: Development of a test to measure gastric accommodation in humans. Am J Physiol 1999;277: G1217–G1221.
74 Gerards C, Leodolter A, Glasbrenner B, Malfertheiner P: The impact of *H. pylori* status on the induction of abdominal pain by rectal barostat in patients with irritable bowel syndrome. Gut 1999;45(suppl 5):A340.

Review Article

Digestive Diseases

Dig Dis 2001;19:240–243

Treatment Options for Functional Dyspepsia

Nimish Vakil

University of Wisconsin Medical School, Milwaukee, Wisc., USA

Key Words

Non-ulcer dyspepsia · Proton pump inhibitors · *H. pylori*

Abstract

Non-ulcer dyspepsia is a common condition in primary care. The treatment of this condition is still controversial and no single therapy is uniformly effective. In this article we review currently available treatment trials for non-ulcer dyspepsia.

Introduction

Dyspepsia (also called uninvestigated dyspepsia) is defined as pain or discomfort centered in the upper abdomen [1]. Non-ulcer dyspepsia or functional dyspepsia refers to a group of patients who have been investigated to rule out organic causes of dyspepsia. To meet the criteria for the definition of non-ulcer dyspepsia, patients must have had dyspeptic symptoms for at least 12 weeks within the preceding 12 months of: (1) persistent or recurrent dyspepsia (as defined above); (2) no evidence of organic disease (including upper endoscopy) that is likely to explain the symptoms, and (3) no evidence that the dyspepsia is exclusively relieved by defecation or associated with the onset of a change in stool frequency or stool form (i.e. not irritable bowel syndrome) [1].

The minimum work-up for a diagnosis of functional dyspepsia is a careful history, physical examination and upper endoscopy during a symptomatic period off antisecretory therapy.

Problems with Therapeutic Trials in Functional Dyspepsia

Treatment studies in non-ulcer dyspepsia have had many methodologic weaknesses. There is a high placebo response rate and therefore adequate controls are essential to allow appropriate comparisons. As there are no objective findings to evaluate at endoscopy, symptom scales are used to assess response. Scales need to be validated to ensure their responsiveness and test-retest reliability. Blinding of patients and controls is critical to prevent bias and a prolonged follow-up is necessary to determine if the effects are truly sustained. Many trials have lacked critical elements in the design that make the results difficult to interpret.

Treatment Strategies in Non-Ulcer Dyspepsia

Helicobacter pylori *Eradication Therapy*

The discovery of *H. pylori* infection opened a new chapter in the treatment of non-ulcer dyspepsia. *H. pylori* infection causes chronic gastritis and it is therefore rea-

KARGER

Fax + 41 61 306 12 34
E-Mail karger@karger.ch
www.karger.com

0257–2753/01/0193–0240$17.50/0

Accessible online at:
www.karger.com/journals/ddi

Nimish Vakil, MD
University of Wisconsin Medical School, Aurora Sinai Medical Center
945 North 12th Street, Room 4040
Milwaukee, WI 53233 (USA)
Tel. +1 414 219 7762, Fax +1 414 219 7108, E-Mail nvakil@facstaff.wisc.edu

sonable to consider eradication therapy. Early trials were improperly controlled, lacked blinding and yielded contradictory results that were difficult to interpret because of the weakness in methodology. More recently a number of well-designed randomized controlled trials have been reported that address the issue of *H. pylori* eradication in non-ulcer dyspepsia. Two recent meta-analyses also evaluate the question of therapy in this setting. Unfortunately, there is still no consensus on the efficacy of *H. pylori* eradication in non-ulcer dyspepsia although it is clear that the majority of patients do not benefit.

Randomized Controlled Trials of H. pylori *Eradication in Non-Ulcer Dyspepsia*

There are four double-blind, randomized, placebo-controlled trials of adequate size that evaluate the efficacy of *H. pylori* eradication in non-ulcer dyspepsia. The design of these studies addresses many of the weaknesses of earlier trials but conflicting results have been reported in them.

Blum et al. [2] randomly assigned 438 patients with *H. pylori* infection and non-ulcer dyspepsia to proton pump inhibitor (PPI) triple therapy or omeprazole alone for 1 week and followed patients for 1 year using validated symptom scales. Treatment success was reported in 27% of patients in the triple therapy group and 21% of patients in the placebo group (not significant). Talley et al. [3] randomly treated 278 infected patients with non-ulcer dyspepsia with PPI triple therapy for 1 week or placebo for 1 week. Relief of dyspepsia at 1 year was similar in the two groups (24% in active treatment and 22% in placebo). A large, multicenter US trial also showed no benefit for *H. pylori* eradication in non-ulcer dyspepsia [4]. 337 patients with *H. pylori* infection and non-ulcer dyspepsia were randomized to *H. pylori* eradication therapy or matched placebo and followed for 1 year. There was no significant difference in treatment success (defined as minimal or no symptoms of dyspepsia) rates in the active treatment group (46%) and placebo (50%). If a more stringent endpoint of no dyspepsia was considered, 28% of patients on triple therapy compared with 23% on placebo had no symptoms at 12 months by intent-to-treat analysis. There was no significant association between the symptom complex (ulcer-like, reflux-like or dysmotility-like) and the outcome, and there was no correlation in the symptoms with improvement in chronic gastritis at 12 months. An important aspect of this trial was that exit endoscopy was performed in all patients at the end of the study. This provides an assessment of the background prevalence of peptic ulcer disease in the community. In the placebo group the rates for ulcer disease were low (4% duodenal ulcer and 2% gastric ulcer). This is an important finding because it suggests that the number of patients with occult ulcer disease in this population was quite small. In contrast to the studies quoted above, a single-center study from Scotland reported a significant benefit with eradication therapy. McColl et al. [5] treated infected patients with functional dyspepsia with PPI triple therapy or omeprazole for 14 days and followed patients for 1 year. They reported that symptoms resolved in a significantly greater proportion of patients (21%) with *H. pylori* triple therapy than in the placebo group (7%). This study has been evaluated in great detail because the results are different from the other randomized controlled trials. The inclusion criteria in this study permitted patients with heartburn to enter the trial while predominant symptoms of reflux disease were exclusionary in the other trials. A significant proportion of patients in this trial had symptoms of reflux disease. This may account for the low placebo response rate seen in this trial. Cure of dyspepsia in the PPI treatment group was similar to that reported in other European studies (approx. 20%) but the low placebo response may have resulted in a significant result. Another possibility is that the baseline prevalence of *H. pylori*-related ulcer disease is very high in Scotland. In an earlier study of dyspeptic patients in Scotland the same authors found ulcer disease in 40% of 182 *H. pylori*-infected dyspeptic patients in their population. When the prevalence of *H. pylori*-related ulcer disease in a population is high, there is an increased likelihood of including patients with healed peptic ulcer disease in a trial of non-ulcer dyspepsia. These patients are more likely to demonstrate a long-term response to eradication therapy. As the patients were not subjected to endoscopy at the end of the trial as in the US study, we cannot determine with precision the rates of ulcer disease in the placebo group.

Two recent studies are still available only in abstract form. The FROSCH trial from Germany and Switzerland randomized 180 patients with non-ulcer dyspepsia and *H. pylori* infection to omeprazole and amoxicillin or omeprazole for 14 days and followed them for 6 months [6]. The principal outcome measure was defined as follows: no need for further therapy or investigations in the last 3 months of the trial. There was no significant difference between the study groups. A small study from Japan randomized patients to omeprazole, amoxicillin and clarithromycin therapy (n = 50) and 40 patients to omeprazole twice daily with matched placebos [7]. Gastritis improved with eradication therapy but dyspeptic symptoms did not change. The ELAN study is a large randomized controlled

European trial of *H. pylori* eradication [8]. A preliminary report of this trial suggested that if patients were classified as responders (dyspepsia score of 1) or nonresponders, there was a higher proportion of responders (44%) in patients with successful eradication compared to patients without eradication (36%).

Meta-Analyses of H. pylori *Eradication in Non-Ulcer Dyspepsia*

A number of meta-analyses have been performed and some have been criticized for the inclusion and exclusion criteria. Two recent studies are of interest because they have reached opposite conclusions. One recent meta-analysis has suggested that eradication therapy may have modest benefit with 1 responder for every 15 patients treated [9]. The authors found 9 studies that met their inclusion criteria, including the ELAN study mentioned above. No significant heterogeneity was found in this analysis. Another recent meta-analysis reached the opposite conclusion suggesting that there is no benefit for eradication therapy [10]. This study found 7 trials that met their inclusion criteria and the authors found significant heterogeneity and noted that this was caused by the Scottish randomized controlled trial described in detail above. The ELAN study was not included in the latter analysis.

Acid Suppressive Therapy

PPIs and H_2 Receptor Antagonists

There have been mixed results with the use of H_2 receptor antagonists in non-ulcer dyspepsia. A recent meta-analysis concluded that there was some benefit but a large number of the studies had to be excluded from the analysis (only 18 of 150 studies met the inclusion criteria [11]). This suggests that many studies have been poorly conducted. The overall results suggest that H_2 receptor antagonists have a modest effect. With cimetidine the therapeutic benefit above placebo was 14% (95% CI 3–24%) and with ranitidine the therapeutic benefit was 33% (95% CI 23–43%). A recent Cochrane review suggested that H_2 receptor antagonists were effective [8 trials generating 1,125 patients; relative risk reduction 30% (95% CI 4–48%)] [12].

Three recent studies evaluated the effectiveness of PPIs in functional dyspepsia. A total of 1,262 patients with functional dyspepsia were enrolled in 2 studies (BOND or OPERA studies) to omeprazole 20 or 10 mg/day or identical placebo for 4 weeks [13]. Complete symptom relief was seen on the last 3 days of therapy in 38% of patients receiving omeprazole 20 mg, 36% in patients receiving omeprazole 10 mg, and 28% on placebo ($p = 0.002$). Symptom relief was similar in patients who were *H. pylori* positive or negative. Similar data have been reported in preliminary form with lansoprazole in a US population. Peura et al. [14] reported complete symptom relief in 44% of patients given lansoprazole 30 mg for 8 weeks compared to 33% of controls given placebo in a trial lasting 8 weeks. The Cochrane review found 4 trials with 1,248 patients and a relative risk reduction of 12% (95% CI 1–24%) [12].

Prokinetic Agents

Prokinetic agents have somewhat better efficacy than cimetidine. One meta-analysis showed that when cisapride was used, improvement over placebo occurred in 36% (95% CI 28–44%) [14]. A Cochrane review found 12 trials with 829 patients with a relative risk reduction of 50% (95% CI 30–65%) but a funnel plot suggested that these results could be due to publication bias alone [12]. Recent concerns about the safety of cisapride have led to its withdrawal from the USA and other countries and limits its use in non-ulcer dyspepsia. Metaclopramide has a modest effect but the relatively high incidence of side effects is a significant disadvantage.

Miscellaneous: 5-HT_3 Antagonists, Hypnotherapy and Simethicone

Recent studies have shown that alosetron reduces postprandial symptoms such as nausea and bloating in functional dyspepsia without altering gastric accommodation or maximal tolerable volume suggesting that 5-HT_3 antagonism may have a role in upper gastrointestinal sensation [15]. Preliminary data also suggest that hypnotherapy may shorten gastric emptying in both normal and dyspeptic subjects and could be of value in therapy [16]. Simethicone has been shown in one study to be superior to cisapride in resolving the symptoms of dyspepsia in the first 2 weeks [17].

In summary, the treatment of non-ulcer dyspepsia is still dissatisfactory. *H. pylori* eradication has a limited role and a modest effect. Antisecretory therapy has a modest effect and prokinetics may be effective as well but selection bias may exaggerate the benefit of prokinetic agents. There are limited data on 5-HT_3 antagonists and hypnotherapy. New treatment approaches are necessary for this common and often chronic condition.

References

1 Talley NJ, Stanghellii V, Heading RC, Koch KL, Malagelada JR, Tytgat GNJ: Functional gastroduodenal disorders. Gut 1999;45(suppl II):1137–1142.

2 Blum AL, Talley NJ, O'Morain C, van Zanten SV, Labenz J, Stolte M, Louw JA, Stubberod A, Theodors A, Sundin M, Bolling-Sternevald E, Junghard O: Lack of effect of treating *Helicobacter pylori* infection in patients with non-ulcer dyspepsia. N Engl J Med 1998;339:1869–1874.

3 Talley NJ, Jenssens J, Lauritsen K, et al: Eradication of *Helicobacter pylori* in functional dyspepsia – Randomized double-blind placebo-controlled trial with 12 months' follow-up. BMJ 1999;318:833–837.

4 Talley NJ, Vakil N, Ballard ED, Fennerty B: Absence of benefit of eradicating *Helicobacter pylori* in patients with non-ulcer dyspepsia. N Engl J Med 1999;341:1106–1111.

5 McColl K, Murray L, El-Omar E, Dickson A, El-Nujumi A, Wirz A, Kelman A, Penny C, Knill-Jones R, Hilditch T: Symptomatic benefit from eradicating *H. pylori* in patients with non-ulcer dyspepsia. N Engl J Med 1998;339:1869–1874.

6 Koelz HR, Arnold R, Stolte M, Blum AL: Treatment of *Helicobacter pylori* does not improve symptoms of functional dyspepsia. Gastroenterology 1998;114:A182.

7 Miwa H, Hirai S, Nagahara A, et al: Cure of *H. pylori* infection does not improve symptoms in non-ulcer dyspepsia patients: A double-blind placebo-controlled study. Aliment Pharmacol Ther 2000;14:317–324.

8 Malfertheiner P, Fischbach W, Layer P, Moessner J, Stolte M, Leodolter A, Demleitner K, Am Fuchs W: ELAN study proves symptomatic benefit of *Helicobacter pylori* eradication in functional dyspepsia. Gastroenterology 2000;118:A440.

9 Moayyedi P, Soo S, Deeks J, Forman D, Mason J, Innes M, Delaney B: Systematic review and economic evaluation of *Helicobacter pylori* eradication treatment for non-ulcer dyspepsia. BMJ 2000;321:659–664.

10 Laine L, Schoenfeld P, Fennerty MB: *H. pylori* therapy is not effective for treatment of non-ulcer dyspepsia: Meta-analysis of randomized controlled trials. Ann Intern Med 2001;134:361–369.

11 Finney JS, Kinnersley N, Hughes M, Bryan-Tear C, Lothian J: Meta-analysis of anti-secretory and gastrokinetic compounds in functional dyspepsia. J Clin Gastroenterol 1998;26:312–320.

12 Soo S: Pharmacological Interventions for non-ulcer dyspepsia. Cochrane Database Syst Rev 2000;2:CD001960.

13 Talley N, Meineche-Schmidt V, Pare P, Duckworth M, Raisanen P, Pap A, Kordecki H, Schmid V: Effect of omeprazole in functional dyspepsia: Double-blind, randomized, placebo-controlled trials (the Bond and Opera studies). Aliment Pharmacol Ther 1998;12:1055–1065.

14 Peura D, Kovacs T, Metz D, Gudmundson J, Pilmer B: Low-dose lansoprazole: Effective for non-ulcer dyspepsia (abstract). Gastroenterology 2000;118:A439.

15 Kuo B, Camilleri M, Burton D, Viramontes B, McKinzie S, Thomforde G, O'Connor M, Brinkman B: 5-HT_3 antagonism of upper gastrointestinal symptoms after a dyspepsia inducing meal. Gastroenterology 2001;120:A134.

16 Chiarioni G, Benini L, Bonfante F, Menegotti M, Salandini L, Vantini I: Prokinetic effect of a single session of gut oriented hypnotherapy on gastric emptying in normal subjects and dyspeptic patients. Gastroenterology 2001;120:A133.

17 Holtmann G: Randomized double-blind comparison of simethicone with cisapride in functional dyspepsia. Aliment Pharmacol Ther 1999;13:1459–1465.

Review Article

Digestive Diseases

Dig Dis 2001;19:244–250

Update in the Therapeutic Management of Irritable Bowel Syndrome

Augusto Villanueva[a] J. Enrique Domínguez-Muñoz[a] Fermín Mearin[b]

Departments of Gastroenterology, [a]University Hospital of Santiago de Compostela and [b]Vall d'Hebron Hospital, Barcelona, Spain

Key Words

Dietary fiber · Diet · Brain-gut axis · Antidiarrheal agents · Antispasmodic agents · Psychotherapy · Prokinetic agents · Antidepressant agents · Analgesics · Serotonin receptor agonists · Serotonin receptor antagonists

Abstract

Irritable bowel syndrome (IBS) is a remarkably frequent disorder that leads to relevant impairment in patients' quality of life. Four mechanisms are involved in the pathogenesis of IBS: altered intestinal motility; increased visceral sensitivity; disturbed intestinal reflexes (intrinsic and extrinsic), and psychological disorders. The close relationship between the central nervous system and the enteric nervous system (the brain-gut axis) is the basis of the actual research on IBS therapy. It is conceivable that in the near future a better understanding of IBS pathophysiology will help us to tailor treatment for different IBS patients. At the moment, the subclassification of the diverse patterns of symptomatology allows the adjustment of treatments for IBS according to the clinical predominance of each patient. Dietary modifications like fiber supplementation, antidiarrheal agents and antispasmodic drugs are the basis of the current treatment of IBS and depend on the predominant symptom (constipation, diarrhea or pain, respectively). If severe pain is present, antidepressant agents are an appropriate alternative. However, the scientific evidence supporting this current therapeutic approach is limited. Visceral analgesics and serotonin agonists and antagonists may play an important therapeutic role in the near future. However, it is not likely that one single treatment will help every IBS patient and many of them will need a more complex approach with multidisciplinary therapy (diet, psychotherapy, medications).

Irritable bowel syndrome (IBS) is a functional disorder that represents the most frequent diagnosis in gastroenterology. IBS prevalence varies enormously depending on the diagnostic criteria employed for diagnosis [1], but recent epidemiological studies performed in our country have shown that, according to the Rome I criteria, the prevalence of the disease may be as high as 12–14% [1, 2]. However, many patients suffering from IBS never ask for medical assistance so what gastroenterologists see is probably only the tip of the iceberg.

Accurate diagnosis and therapy of IBS will be the result of the evolution in the pathophysiological knowledge achieved over the last decades. At the moment, there is no biological marker for IBS and so far there is no imaging procedure allowing a definite diagnosis of the syndrome. It is conceivable that functional disorders of the gastrointestinal tract have their basis on molecular alterations with no macroscopic correlation explaining why the

KARGER

Fax +41 61 306 12 34
E-Mail karger@karger.ch
www.karger.com

0257–2753/01/0193–0244$17.50/0

Accessible online at:
www.karger.com/journals/ddi

J. Enrique Domínguez-Muñoz
Department of Gastroenterology
University Hospital, C/ Choupana s/n
E–15706 Santiago de Compostela (Spain)
Tel. +34 981 950 070, Fax +34 981 951 378, E-Mail jdominguezm@medynet.com

search for pathological findings to achieve the diagnosis is difficult. Nowadays, the diagnosis of IBS is based on clinical findings. Clinical criteria for IBS diagnosis have changed over the last two decades. From the Manning criteria [3] to the Rome II criteria [4] changes were made with the intention of increasing the sensitivity and mainly the specificity in order to restrict IBS diagnosis and permit the development of clinical trials and studies on the natural history of the disease [5]. The first step in the diagnosis of IBS is the exclusion of any organic disease explaining symptoms. The thoroughness of this evaluation will mainly depend on clinical suspicion, evolution time and patient age. Thus, it is recommended that at least patients older than 40 years and those with alarm symptoms undergo some exploration of the colon to avoid misdiagnosis of organic disorders [6].

The clinical features of IBS include abdominal pain and alterations in the patient's bowel movement habits. In the last decade, morbidity associated with these symptoms has been studied by means of quality-of-life scales. Like other diseases which disturb life activities, IBS is accompanied by a sphere of biopsychosocial implications. The WHO introduced the concepts of disability, impairment and handicap to accurately define the impact of diseases on quality of life so that the differently designed scales fulfil all aspects of life restrictions caused by diseases. Impairment is defined as the signs and symptoms that are a direct consequence of the disease. Disability is the boundary or the loss of ability to perform activities that would be considered normal for a human being (limitations of daily activities caused by disease). Handicap represents the effects of the disease in terms of restricting the patient's development in society (social and environmental limitations because of disease) [7]. The impact of IBS includes every aspect of life (sleep, sexual activity, diet, work, etc.) and therefore there is an important disability, impairment and handicap caused by IBS that should be measured by means of quality-of-life scales. This allows the evaluation of patterns of evolution of the disease and the analysis of therapeutic assays. Most scales focus on the same items (emotional health, physical functioning, avoidance of food, fatigue, anxiety, etc.) [8–11] and are an extremely useful tool for the evaluation of new drugs on IBS treatment.

At the beginning of this century it is though that there are four main mechanisms implicated in the pathophysiology of IBS: altered intestinal motility; increased visceral sensitivity; disturbed intestinal reflexes (intrinsic and extrinsic), and psychological disorders (fig. 1). The predominance and combination of these mechanisms are most probably responsible for the different manifestations and subgroups of IBS (i.e. diarrhea-predominant, constipation-predominant or pain-predominant IBS).

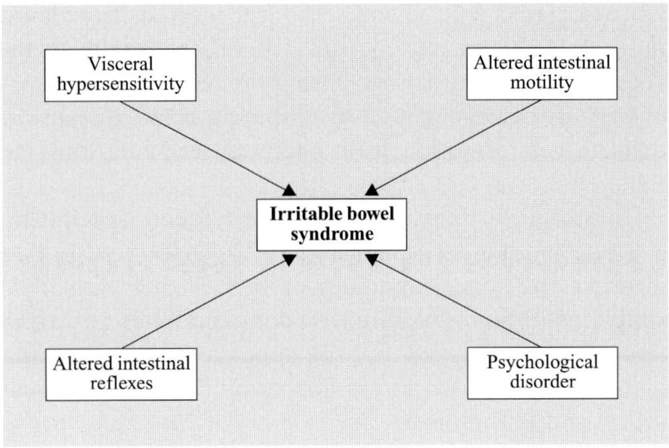

Fig. 1. Mechanisms implicated in the pathophysiology of irritable bowel syndrome. These alterations are the therapeutic targets for the management of this syndrome.

Non-Pharmacological Therapies

Diet

As a first step in the management of IBS patients, the avoidance of nutrients that will probably induce symptoms (i.e. voluminous meals, fat, nonabsorbable carbohydrates, coffee, tea, lactose) is frequently recommended. However, there is no scientific evidence supporting this approach and one should never forget the main goal of maintaining an adequate quality of life for IBS patients that can be considerably limited by restricting the usual dietary habits.

Clinical trials evaluating diet modifications have been centered on pain relief and changes in stool characteristics. Most placebo-controlled trials were performed with fiber. A fiber-enriched diet (20–30 g/day) improves constipation, accelerates intestinal transit and may reduce intracolonic pressure [12]. Furthermore, fiber is associated with a reduction in the intracolonic concentration of bile acids, which may reduce the contractile activity of the colon [13, 14]. However, patients with IBS do not have less fiber intake than asymptomatic control subjects [12]. In addition, clinical trials have not found any significant benefit of a fiber-enriched diet compared to placebo [15]. The symptomatic improvement found in these trials was not associated with changes in fecal mass or in colonic motility [15]. Last but not least, fiber therapy may aggravate IBS symptoms by decreasing the pain threshold secondary to distension and by inducing colon distension through gas formation from bacterial fermentation [16, 17].

In summary, there is no scientific evidence supporting the idea that standard changes in dietary habits or lifestyle improve the symptomatology of IBS. A diet with fiber supplementation could improve constipation in constipation-predominant IBS, but the appearance or worsening of symptoms related to gas formation limits the clinical utility of this approach.

Psychotherapy

It seems evident from clinical practice that psychological factors play a significant role in IBS manifestations. Recently the close relationship between the central nervous system and the gastrointestinal tract (particularly the enteric nervous system) has been described and coined as the 'brain-gut axis'. Patients with IBS frequently have psychological complaints associated with digestive disorders but it is difficult to know which is the cause and which the consequence.

Another important point is the fear of having a malignant disease, since around 60% of IBS patients compared to only 30% of those with organic disease are afraid of having cancer. Unfortunately, only 29% of them lose their fear of having a malignant disease after visiting the doctor [18].

The clinical response to psychotherapy is limited and very often restricted because of the lack of availability in daily practice. Moreover, not every patient profits from this intervention [19]. However, if psychotherapy is not available or not indicated for a given patient, profound explanation of the syndrome by the doctor is mandatory to improve coping and avoid unnecessary fear. At least it may be clear that IBS is not a malignant disease and that it is not a risk factor for cancer, but a chronic syndrome which is difficult to treat.

Pharmacological Therapies

Antidiarrheal Drugs

Loperamide is the most widely used drug for diarrhea-predominant IBS. It is a synthetic opioid, obtained from the basis of meperidine, with no effect on the central nervous system. Loperamide increases water and ion absorption, decreases intestinal transit time and increases anal sphincter tone [20]. Most of the trials with loperamide on diarrhea-predominant IBS proved beneficial compared to placebo. In a 13-week double-blind placebo-controlled trial loperamide significantly improved stool frequency, consistency and urgency [21]. Another double-blind study confirmed these results but also revealed an increase in nocturnal pain in patients treated with loperamide [22]. The clinical relevance of both trials is limited by the high proportion of dropouts (19 and 30%, respectively). The most important side effects of loperamide are dystonic reactions, although this problem is more frequent in children.

In summary, the present clinical evidence for loperamide in the treatment of IBS is limited and further trials are required. Furthermore, when diarrhea is the predominant symptom in a patient with suspected IBS it is especially important to rule out other potential causes of diarrhea, in particular those related to malabsorption of nutrients and biliary acids, before starting any pharmacological therapy.

Antispasmodic Drugs

The use of antispasmodics with anticholinergic activity is very common in the management of IBS. Several drugs have been evaluated but most trials underwent strong criticisms because of methodological limitations (i.e. low number of patients, large amount of dropouts, short duration of the trials, etc.) and most of them revealed a reliable response to placebo. In fact, among 36 placebo-controlled, double-blind, randomized clinical trials with antispasmodics lasting for more than 2 weeks published to date, only 15 evaluated pain or general symptomatic improvement as an end point. Only 8 trials lasted for at least 6 weeks. Furthermore, the proportion of dropouts was as high as up to 59%. Finally, the placebo response ranged from 23 to 87%, with a mean value of 68%. With these methodological limitations, conclusions on the efficacy of antispasmodics for IBS treatment is at least debatable.

Among the trials mentioned above, 26 were comparable from a methodological point of view and were included by Poynard et al. [23] in a meta-analysis. As a result of this analysis, antispasmodics were found to be superior to placebo in terms of global improvement (62 vs. 35%, $p < 0.01$) and abdominal pain relief (64 vs. 45%, $p < 0.01$). These positive results were obtained with five different drugs: cimetropium bromide, pinaverium bromide, octylonium bromide, trimebutine and mebeverine [23].

Although this family of drugs is widely used in pain-predominant IBS, the available scientific evidence is far from being conclusive and new clinical trials are required. Furthermore, these drugs are not available in every country.

Prokinetic Drugs

To date, the use of prokinetic drugs in IBS has mostly been restricted to cisapride. Cisapride is a benzamide derivative with cholinergic activity in the myoenteric plexus through serotonin-mediated effects (5-HT_4 agonism). There are two double-blind trials with 5–10 mg of cisapride on IBS [24, 25]. No significant differences were found between placebo and cisapride, with the exception of stool passage (which improved with the drug) in one of the trials [25]. These results limit cisapride use in IBS to patients with remarkable functional symptomatology of the upper gastrointestinal tract. Moreover, restriction in the use of cisapride due to cardiac side effect makes this drug inappropriate for standard IBS treatment.

Psychodrugs

The use of psychotropic drugs in IBS is based upon two concepts: one is the fact that IBS patients, as mentioned above, have an outstanding psychological profile, so antidepressant drugs could play a role in the central nervous component of the syndrome. On the other hand, most psychotropic agents have a mechanism of action through molecules implicated in neural synapses. Thus, tricyclic antidepressants have an analgesic effect mediated by ion channel blockers [26] and this effect is obtained at doses lower than that required for depression therapy. The main advantage achieved with this kind of drug is, therefore, pain relief in diarrhea-predominant IBS. A trial with desipramine demonstrated a significant decrease in stool frequency, abdominal pain and depression, compared to placebo and atropine [27]. Similar results were obtained in another study using trimipramine [28]. However, it must be taken into account that these drugs may have important side effects that can limit its use in many patients (i.e. urinary retention, xerostomia, etc.) leading even to death in cases of overdose because of heart-related toxicity.

In conclusion, patients with IBS may benefit from antidepressant drugs, especially tricyclic antidepressants, at low doses. This is especially true in patients with severe pain who do not respond to first-line therapies, have intense limitations in activities of daily life, have diarrhea predominance, and/or have depression linked to IBS.

Visceral Analgesics

Based on the new pathophysiological concepts of IBS, therapeutic research focuses on new molecules able to modulate the visceral perception of the gastrointestinal tract. Fedotozine, an opioid analog with selective kappa receptor affinity, has been evaluated in the treatment of IBS patients. A trial performed with fedotozine (3.5, 15 and 30 mg) revealed that the 30 mg group was significantly superior to placebo in controlling abdominal pain, abdominal bloating and global severity of the disease [29]. Nevertheless, due to its marginal clinical benefit and putative secondary effects it does not seem that fedotozine will be available for clinical use.

Some other drugs such as octreotide (a somatostatin analog) and leuprolide (a gastrin-releasing hormone analog) might also improve abdominal pain in some IBS patients. Clonidine, an α_2-adrenergic agonist, decreases pain sensation during colonic distension and increases rectal compliance in healthy controls and IBS patients. However, several problems (i.e. administration route, secondary effects) preclude its clinical application.

The Serotoninergic System

Over the last decades there has been an increased interest in treating IBS patients according to the newest pathophysiological concepts. In this context, the role of serotonin in the enteric nervous system has become one of the most important sources of molecules. Serotonin was first isolated in 1952 in the enterochromaffin tissue of the gut. Around 95% of the total quantity of serotonin is located in the gastrointestinal tract, and only 5% in the central nervous system. Serotonin production and secretion in the gastrointestinal tract is mediated by very different stimuli, among them chemical (i.e. gastrin) and mechanical (i.e. distension of the gut) stimuli are the most important. There are at least four subtypes of serotonin receptors: 5-HT_1 and 5-HT_2 are located mostly in the central nervous system, while 5-HT_3 and 5-HT_4 develop their functions in the gastrointestinal tract (although recently it has been found that other receptor subtypes appear to play a promising role in IBS pathophysiology, like 5-HT_7 and $5\text{-HT}_{1B/D}$).

Two different pathways related to serotonin exist in the enteric nervous system with different behavior after stimulation. The intrinsic pathway (mainly mediated through 5-HT_4 receptors) is involved in the peristaltic reflexes and the secretion of water and ions, Cl^- being the most significant. The extrinsic pathway (mainly mediated by 5-HT_3 receptors) is associated with visceral sensations (nausea, meteorism, pain, etc.). Both mechanisms implicated in IBS manifestations, visceral hypersensitivity (exaggerated experience of pain in response to physiological stimuli) [30] and motility alterations, are controlled, at least in part, by serotonin.

Serotonin Antagonists

There is a clinical model of serotonin actions in the gastrointestinal tract: the carcinoid syndrome. The diarrhea associated with this syndrome is related to serotonin overproduction, which causes motor and secretory hyperstimulation of the gastrointestinal tract. Based on this, several clinical trials were carried out in order to test the usefulness of serotonin antagonists in the treatment of IBS, especially diarrhea-predominant IBS. A double-blind pilot study with ondansetron (a 5-HT_3-specific blocker) versus placebo in 14 patients with diarrhea-predominant IBS revealed no significant differences in terms of colonic transit modification between both groups, although there were 11 dropouts in this study [31]. Another double-blind study performed in 1996 with ondansetron versus placebo proved a significant decrease in abdominal distension and the frequency of abdominal pain compared with placebo [32]. Maxton et al. [33] performed a similar placebo-controlled trial with ondansetron including 50 patients and demonstrated a significant reduction in the frequency of bowel movements and an increase in stool consistency in those with diarrhea-predominant IBS [33].

The most evaluated 5-HT_3-selective antagonist in IBS is alosetron, which proved its capacity to decrease colonic transit and to increase jejunal absorption of water and sodium. A trial performed in 647 non-constipated women with IBS and focusing on abdominal pain showed improvement in 41% of patients receiving alosetron versus 29% receiving placebo [34]. A similar study with 462 patients had equivalent results with significant differences for alosetron versus placebo in decreasing the score for diarrhea and increasing the number of days free from pain [35]. A recent study also demonstrated that alosetron significantly improves health-related quality of life in women with IBS, especially in patients with diarrhea-predominant IBS [36]. A comparison of alosetron with two antispasmodic drugs (mebeverine and trimebutine) also showed significant differences in favor of alosetron in controlling IBS-related symptomatology [37]. These findings made alosetron the first Food and Drug Administration-approved agent for diarrhea-predominant IBS. However, significant side effects have been noted with the use of this drug, including intense constipation and fecal impaction. Moreover, some cases of ischemic colitis were detected, but some of the patients recovered after interrupting the drug [38]. Because of this, the Food and Drug Administration withdrew their approval for alosetron. In March 2001 the results of a study on the tolerability and safety of alosetron in 859 patients were reported with no deaths related to the study drug, and constipation being the most frequent adverse effect (typically during the first month of treatment) [39]. A second-generation 5-HT_4-receptor antagonist is under evaluation for the treatment of diarrhea-predominant IBS.

Serotonin Agonists

Tegaserod is a partial agonist of 5-HT_4 receptors with a prokinetic effect on gastric emptying and is able to increase colonic and bowel transit. It stimulates intestinal secretion of water and Cl^-, and decreases the response to rectal distension [40]. Tegaserod was meant to be a drug for constipation-predominant IBS and several trials have demonstrated a significant reduction in abdominal pain and an increase in bowel movement frequency mediated by this drug [41]. So far there have been no serious adverse effects related to the use of this drug.

Treatment of Bacterial Overgrowth

A recent study found that treatment of bacterial overgrowth in patients with IBS results in elimination of the IBS criteria used in the design of the study [42]. The relation between IBS and bacterial overgrowth is not yet fully established but opens a door for further subclassifications of the disease.

Conclusions

The close relationship between the central nervous system and the enteric nervous system (the brain-gut axis) is the basis of the actual research on IBS, not only concerning pathophysiology but also treatment. Whether therapy has to be aimed at the gut, the neural pathways controlling bowel motility and perception, or the processing mechanisms of symptoms and disease behavior is still unclear. It is conceivable that in the near future better understanding of IBS pathophysiology will help us to tailor treatment for different IBS patients. At the moment, subclassification of the diverse patterns of symptomatology allows adjustment of new treatments for IBS according to the clinical predominance for each patient (fig. 2). The knowledge of motor and sensorial responses to different stimuli in IBS patients and the pathways to the central nervous system is an important source of information for the development

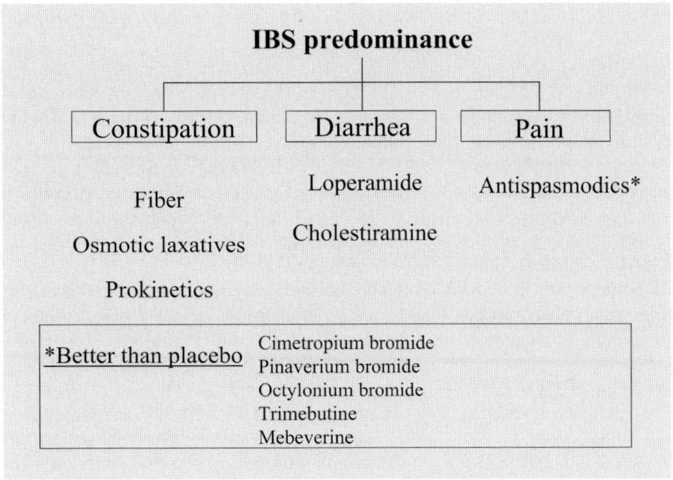

Fig. 2. Symptomatic therapies for irritable bowel syndrome (IBS) according to the predominant symptom.

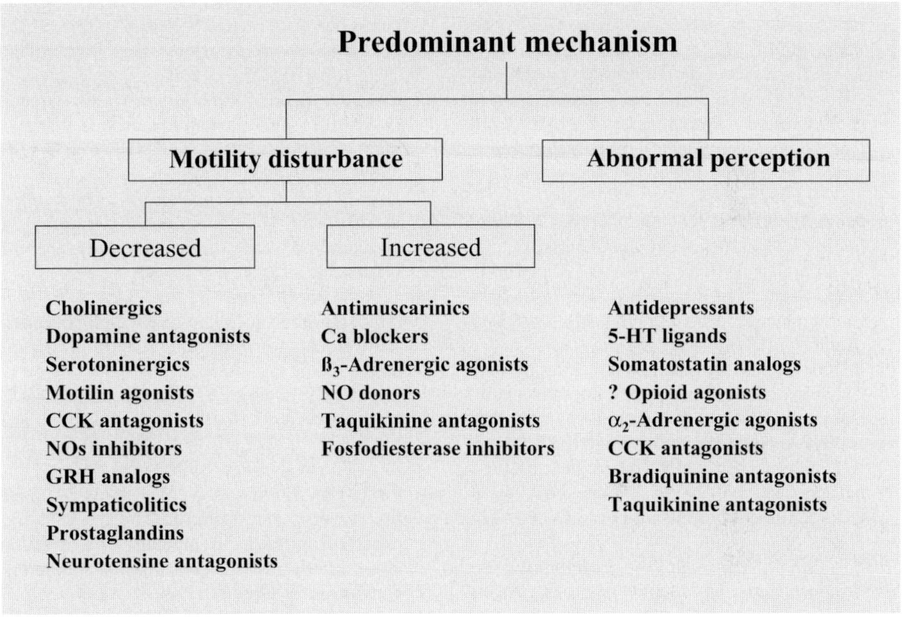

Fig. 3. Pathophysiological therapy of irritable bowel syndrome according to the predominant mechanism of disease.

of new molecules. Furthermore since IBS is a disease with relevant impact on the patients' quality of life, evaluation of the psychological burden related to the disease is an important tool for the treatment of this disease. A fiber-enriched diet is frequently given for constipation-predominant IBS. Loperamide, antispasmodic drugs and tricyclic antidepressants are nowadays the basis of pharmacological treatment. The scientific evidence supporting this therapeutic approach is, however, limited. Visceral analgesics and serotonin agonists and antagonists may play an important therapeutic role in the near future. The study of the most probable mechanism of disease in each patient may lead to a more adequate therapeutic approach (fig. 3). However, it is not likely that one single treatment will help every IBS patient and many of them will need a more complex approach with a multidisciplinary therapy (diet, psychotherapy, medications). The complexity and diversity are key points in IBS.

References

1 Meearin F, Badía X, Balboa A, Baró E, Caldwell E, Cucala M, Díaz-Rubio M, Fueyo A, Ponce J, Roset M, Talley NJ: Irritable bowel syndrome prevalence varies enormously depending on the employed diagnostic criteria: Comparisons of Rome II versus previous criteria in a general population. Scand J Gastroenterol, in press.

2 Caballero-Plasencia AM, Sofos-Kontoyannis S, Valenzuela-Barranco M, Martin-Ruiz JL, López-Manas JG: Irritable bowel syndrome in patients with dyspepsia. A community-based study in southern Europe. Eur J Gastroenterol Hepatol 1999;11:517–522.

3 Manning AP, Thompson WG, Heaton KW, Morris AF: Towards a positive diagnosis of the irritable bowel. Br Med J 1978;ii:653–654.

4 Drossman DA, Corazziari E, Talley NJ, Thompson WG, Whitehead WE: Rome II: A multinational consensus document on functional gastrointestinal disorders. Gut 1999; 45(suppl 2):1–81.

5 Saito YA, Locke GR, Talley NJ, Zinsmeister AR, Fett SL, Melton LJ 3rd: A comparison of the Rome and Manning criteria for case identification in epidemiological investigations of irritable bowel syndrome. Am J Gastroenterol 2000;95:2679–2681.

6 Jones J, Boorman J, Cann P, Forbes A, Gomborone J, Heaton K, Hungin P, Kumar D, Libby G, Spiller R, Read N, Silk D, Whorwell P: British Society of Gastroenterology guidelines for the management of the irritable bowel syndrome. Gut 2000;47(suppl 2):ii1–19.

7 World Health Organization: International Classification of Impairments, Disabilities and Handicaps. Geneva, WHO, 1980.

8 Hahn BA, Kirchdoerfer LJ, Fullerton S, Mayer E: Evaluation of a new quality of life questionnaire for patients with irritable bowel syndrome. Aliment Pharmacol Ther 1997;11:547–552.

9 Patrick DL, Drossman DA, Frederick IO, DiCesare J, Puder KL: Quality of life in persons with irritable bowel syndrome: Development and validation of a new measure. Dig Dis Sci 1998;43:400–411.

10 Wong E, Guyatt GH, Cook DJ, Griffith LE, Irvine EJ: Development of a questionnaire to measure quality of life in patients with irritable bowel syndrome. Eur J Surg 1998;583(suppl): 50–56.

11 Chassany O, Marquis P, Scherrer B, Read NW, Finger T, Bergmann JF, Fraitag B, Geneve J, Caulin C: Validation of a specific quality of life questionnaire for functional digestive disorders. Gut 1999;44:527–533.

12 Cann PA, Read NM, Holdsworth CD: What is the benefit of coarse wheat bran in patients with irritable bowel syndrome? Gut 1984;25: 168–173.

13 Snook J, Shepherd HA: Bran supplementation in the treatment of irritable bowel syndrome. Aliment Pharmacol Ther 1994;8:511–514.

14 Muller-Lissner SA: Effect of wheat bran on weight of stool and gastrointestinal transit time: A meta-analysis. Br Med J (Clin Res Ed) 1988;296:615–617.

15 Lucey MR, Clarck ML, Lowndes J, Dawson AM: Is bran efficacious in irritable bowel syndrome? A double-blind, placebo-controlled crossover study. Gut 1987;28:221–225.

16 Whitehead WE, Holtkotter B, Enck P, Hoelzl R, Holmes KD, Anthony J, Shabsin HS, Schuster MM: Tolerance for rectosigmoid distension in irritable bowel syndrome. Gastroenterology 1990;98:1187–1192.

17 Haderstorfer B, Psycholgin D, Whitehead WE, Schuster MM: Intestinal gas production from bacterial fermentation of undigested carbohydrate in irritable bowel syndrome. Am J Gastroenterol 1989;84:375–378.

18 Thompson WG, Lonstreth GF, Drossman DA, Heaton KW, Irvine EJ, Muller-Lissner SA: Functional bowel disorders and functional abdominal pain. Gut 1999;45(suppl 2):II43–47.

19 Guthrie E, Creed F, Dawson D, Tomerson B: A controlled trial of psychological treatment for the irritable bowel syndrome. Gastroenterology 1991;100:450–457.

20 Cann PA, Read NW, Holdsworth CD, Barends D: Role of loperamide and placebo in management of irritable bowel syndrome. Dig Dis Sci 1984;29:239–247.

21 Lavo B, Stenstam M, Nielsen AL: Loperamide in treatment of irritable bowel syndrome, a double-blind placebo controlled study. Scand J Gastroenterol 1987;130:77–80.

22 Efskind PS, Bernklev T, Vatn MH: A double-blind, placebo-controlled trial with loperamide in irritable bowel syndrome. Scand J Gastroenterol 1996;31:463–468.

23 Poynard T, Naveau S, Mory B, Chaput JC: Meta-analysis of smooth muscle relaxant in the treatment of irritable bowel syndrome. Aliment Pharmacol Ther 1994;8:499–510.

24 Farup PG, Hovdenak N, Wetterhus S, Lange OJ, Hovde O, Trondstad R: The symptomatic effect of cisapride in patients with irritable bowel syndrome and constipation. Scand J Gastroenterol 1998;33:128–131.

25 Schutze K, Brandstatter G, Dragosics B, Judmaier G, Hentschel E: Double-blind study of the effect of cisapride on constipation and abdominal discomfort as components of the irritable bowel syndrome. Aliment Pharmacol Ther 1997;11:387–394.

26 Gerner P, Mujtaba M, Sinnott CJ, Wang GK: Amitriptyline versus bupivacaine in rat sciatic nerve blockade. Anesthesiology 2001;94:661–667.

27 Greenbaum DS, Mayle JE, Vanegeren LE, Jerome JA, Mayor JW, Greenbaum RB, Matson RW, Stein GE, Dean HA, Halvorsen NA, Rosen LW: The effects of desipramine on IBS compared with atropine and placebo. Dig Dis Sci 1987;32:257–566.

28 Myren J, Lovland B, Larssen SE, Larsen S: A double-blind study of the effect of trimipramine in patients with the irritable bowel syndrome. Scand J Gastroenterol 1984;19:835–843.

29 Dapoigny M, Abitbol JL, Fraitag B: Efficacy of peripheral kappa agonist, fedotozine, vs. placebo in treatment of irritable bowel syndrome. A multicenter dose-response study. Dig Dis Sci 1995;40:2244–2249.

30 Wilhelmsen I: Brain-gut axis as an example of the bio-psycho-social model. Gut 2000;47 (suppl 4):iv5–iv7.

31 Steadman CJ, Talley NJ, Phillips SF, Zinsmeister AR: Selective 5-hydroxytryptamine type 3 receptor antagonism with ondansetron as treatment for diarrhea-predominant irritable bowel syndrome: a pilot study. Mayo Clin Proc 1992;67:732–738.

32 Goldberg PA, Kamm MA, Setti-Carraro P, van der Sijp JR, Roth C: Modification of visceral sensitivity and pain in irritable bowel syndrome by 5-HT_3 antagonism (ondansetron). Digestion 1996:57;478–483.

33 Maxton DG, Morris J, Whorwell PJ: Selective 5-hydroxytryptamine antagonism: A role in irritable bowel syndrome and functional dyspepsia?. Aliment Pharmacol Ther 1996;10:595–599.

34 Camilleri M, Northcutt AR, Kong S, Dukes GE, McSorley D, Mangel AW: Efficacy and safety of alosetron in women with irritable bowel syndrome: A randomised, placebo-controlled trial. Lancet 2000;355:1035–1040.

35 Bardhan KD, Bodemar G, Geldof H, Schutz E, Heath A, Mills JG, Jacques LA: A double-blind, randomized, placebo-controlled dose-ranging study to evaluate the efficacy of alosetron in the treatment of irritable bowel syndrome. Aliment Pharmacol Ther 2000;14:23–34.

36 Watson ME, Lacey L, Kong S, Northcutt AR, McSorley D, Hahn B, Mangel AW: Alosetron improves quality of life in women with diarrhea-predominant irritable bowel syndrome. Am J Gastroenterol 2001;96:455–459.

37 Jones RH, Holtmann G, Rodrigo L, Ehsanullah RS, Crompton PM, Jacques LA, Mills JG: Alosetron relieves pain and improves bowel function compared with mebeverine in female nonconstipated irritable bowel syndrome patients. Aliment Pharcacol Ther 1999;13:1419–1427.

38 Friedel D, Thomas R, Fisher RS: Ischemic colitis during treatment with alosetron. Gastroenterology 2001;120:557–560.

39 Wolfe SG, Chey WY, Washington MK, Harding J, Heath AT, McSorley DJ, Dukes GE, Hunt CM: Tolerability and safety of alosetron during long-term administration in female and male irritable bowel syndrome patients. Am J Gastroenterol 2001;96:803–811.

40 Prather CM, Camilleri M, Zinsmeister AR, McKinzie S, Thomforde G: Tegaserod accelerates orocecal transit in patients with constipation-predominant irritable bowel syndrome. Gastroenterology 2000;118:463–468.

41 De Ponti F, Tonini M: Irritable bowel syndrome: New agents targeting serotonin receptor subtypes. Drugs 2001;61:317–332.

42 Pimentel M, Chow E, Lin HC: Eradication of small intestine bacterial overgrowth reduces symptoms of irritable bowel syndrome. Am J Gastroenterol 2000;95:3503–3506.

Original Paper

Digestive Diseases

Dig Dis 2001;19:251–257

Irritable Bowel Syndrome in Mexico

Ivonne Huerta Miguel Angel Valdovinos Max Schmulson

Department of Gastroenterology, Instituto Nacional de Ciencias Médicas y Nutrición Salvador Zubirán, Mexico City, Mexico

Key Words

Irritable bowel syndrome · Epidemiology · Quality of life · Rome criteria

Abstract

The current review includes all the available original data on irritable bowel syndrome in Mexico. Data were organized in items of interest such as prevalence and gender distribution, health care utilization, psychosocial factors, diagnostic criteria, bowel habit predominance, physiological studies, clinical trials and quality of life assessment. After a systematic review, a total of 18 papers were included, the majority published between 1996 and 2000. We can conclude that irritable bowel syndrome in Mexico is similar to that reported in the international literature with regard to the areas analyzed, and therefore it is suitable to run clinical trials with similar outcomes as has been done in other populations.

Introduction

Irritable bowel syndrome (IBS) is considered the most frequent functional bowel disorder around the world, and for many years there was very little scientific information on its mechanisms, therefore treatment was very limited [1]. The advance in technology to assess gastrointestinal motility and more recently visceral hypersensitivity has led to an increase in the knowledge of the pathophysiological basis of IBS, and ultimately to the development of newer medications [2–4]. These factors have increased the interest of research in the field even more.

Lately this interest has also been rising in Mexico, therefore we sought to determine the status of IBS in this country by conducting a systematic review of all the relevant original literature available.

Methods

Data Sources

All studies which originated in Mexico and were published in the Spanish and/or English languages were identified by a comprehensive electronic search of Medline from 1970 to 2000. A search for the medical subject headings, *irritable bowel syndrome, irritable colon syndrome,* and *functional bowel disorder,* limited by the term, *Mexico*, was done. Furthermore, searches using the limiting terms, *Spanish* and *clinical*, and the Medline abbreviations of all Mexican and Latin gastroenterological journals were also done. This strategy was supplemented by a manual search of the references from all retrieved publications for citations of Mexican authors. Finally, abstracts of known Mexican researchers in the field that were published in Latin and American gastroenterological journals were included.

KARGER

Fax + 41 61 306 12 34
E-Mail karger@karger.ch
www.karger.com

0257–2753/01/0193–0251$17.50/0

Accessible online at:
www.karger.com/journals/ddi

Max Schmulson, MD
Department of Gastroenterology
Instituto Nacional de Ciencias Médicas y Nutrición Salvador Zubirán
Vasco de Quiroga No. 15 Tlalpan, CP 14000 Mexico City (Mexico)
Tel. +52 5 5733418, Fax +52 5 6550942, E-Mail maxjulio@quetzal.innsz.mx

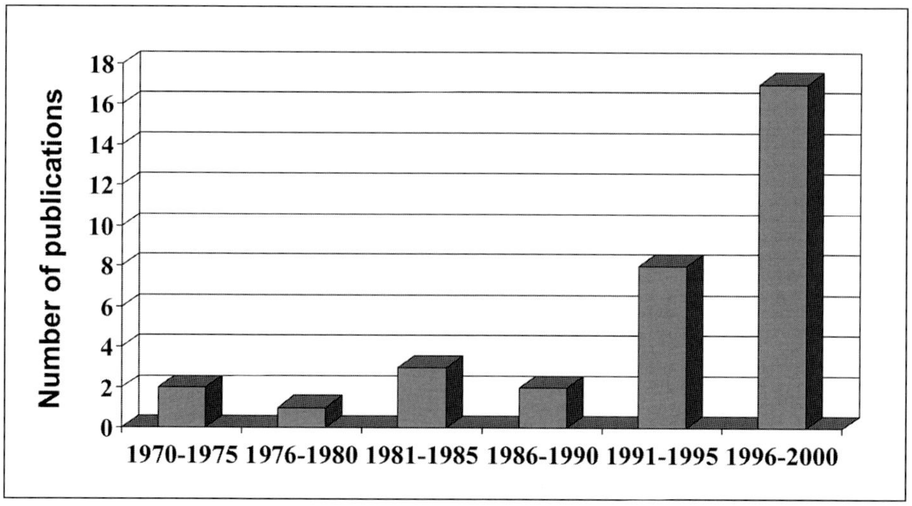

Fig. 1. Number of Mexican publications on IBS over different time periods.

Data Description

Data were organized in items of interest: prevalence and gender distribution; impact of IBS on health care utilization; psychosocial factors; diagnostic criteria; symptom subgroups based on predominant bowel habit; physiological studies; clinical trials, and quality of life assessment. For each item, an introduction of known data was used as the framework for the description of the Mexican data.

Results

A total of 33 publications were identified, the majority published between 1996 and 2000 (fig. 1). Five publications were review articles and thus were excluded [5–9]. Of the original studies, 5 were excluded because they did not address standard diagnostic or physiological criteria [10–15]. Three publications were duplicated because they were published in abstract form as well as in full text, in this case the full text was cited [16–18]. Furthermore, one of these abstracts was published in a local as well as in an international journal [19]. Finally a total of 18 studies were included, 8 published in full text [16–18, 20–24] and 10 in abstract form [25–34]. This information was supplemented by data from an epidemiological study conducted between 1999 and 2000 by the Mexican Gastroenterological Association that has not yet been published, but the results were presented at the national meeting of the same association [34].

Prevalence and Gender Distribution

It is estimated that the prevalence of IBS is similar around the world ranging from 5 to 25% and it is probably independent of genetic, environmental or dietary factors in different populations [35]. In Mexico several small epidemiological studies have been conducted. In 1982 one study reported a 20.4% prevalence of IBS [20]. In another study that was conducted in a random rural population of the center of Mexico using Manning criteria, IBS was found in 8.7 and 20.4% of the 184 males and 309 females included. In the same study, 17% of the males and 28% of the females reported to be devoid of digestive symptoms, and a lower educational level was inversely related to the presence of IBS [26].

Using the Rome I criteria we performed a questionnaire study in Mexico City among 174 students with a mean age of 19.8 years who were studying at a private medical school. The study demonstrated an IBS prevalence of 17.8% with a 4:1 female:male ratio [27]. In another study among 98 IBS patients (based on Rome I criteria) from a tertiary referral center and without any other medical condition, the female:male ratio was 2.5:1.0 [24]. In this study, the mean age of the participants was 40.8 years.

Recently, a study has provided information about the pediatric population in Mexico. Using Rome II criteria, an IBS prevalence of 26.9% was found among pediatric patients, age ranging between 4 and 16 years [32]. Table 1 summarizes the epidemiological characteristics of IBS in Mexico.

Impact of IBS on Health Care Utilization

IBS results in high cost to society, in terms of work absenteeism and use of health care resources [35–37]. In an attempt to determine the frequency of visits to gastroenterologists by IBS patients, the Mexican Gastroentero-

Table 1. Epidemiological characteristics of IBS in Mexico

Prevalence between 18 and 20%
Female to male ratio: 2.4–4.0:1.0
Bowel habit predominance: 50% alternating and the other 50% equally distributed among constipation and diarrhea predominance
Number one cause of consultation of a gastroenterologist
Frequent history of abdominal surgery
Associated with depression and anxiety disorders
Lower quality of life as compared to organic disorders

logical Association conducted a questionnaire study among 1,497 patients from different parts of the country who consulted 37 members of the Association for the first time. It was found that IBS (determined by Rome II) was the primary reason for consultation, accounting for 23% of the initial visits [34].

We have evaluated the use of health care resources in a tertiary referral academic center and reviewed the medical records of 98 IBS patients without any other medical condition [24]. During a mean of 33.4 months of follow-up, a mean of 5 diagnostic studies/patient were ordered prior to IBS diagnosis, and even though in the majority of cases the diagnosis was established during the first medical visit, a mean of 17 studies was ordered afterwards. Each patient consulted a physician an average of 3.6 times/year, 44% of the consultations for gastrointestinal symptoms and 49% for non-gastrointestinal symptoms [24], which was similar to that reported elsewhere [36, 37]. The consultations in the highest demand after internal medicine (53%) and gastroenterology (39%) were proctology (32%), psychiatry (21%), gynecology (18%) and urology (13%). There was a 22- and 2-fold increase in appendectomies and cholecystectomies, respectively, in IBS patients as compared to the total number of hospital discharges for the same period of time. Moreover, most of the surgeries were performed prior to the diagnosis of IBS being established [24].

Psychosocial Factors

The coexistence of psychiatric disorders, mainly depression and anxiety, with IBS has been reported in 42–61% of the patients seen in gastroenterology clinics [38]. It has also been found that IBS patients who seek medical attention have greater psychological disturbances than those who do not seek medical care and controls [39]. Psychological disturbances influence health care-seeking behavior, and psychological stressors such as a history of physical or sexual abuse, major loss and others, influence the development of IBS [1].

Using the Zung scale for depression and the Hamilton scale for anxiety, it was reported in 1982 that patients with functional bowel disorders in a Mexican tertiary referral center had a higher prevalence of depression and anxiety compared to patients with peptic ulcer disease and controls [25]. Recently, in another study that used the Zung self-administered scale that was validated for Mexico, the prevalence of affective disorders among patients with functional gastrointestinal disorders is 80% as compared to 25% in patients without functional gastrointestinal disorders in the same medical center [31]. The most frequent disorders encountered were depression 60% and anxiety 5.4% [31]. In a rural community, a questionnaire study conducted among 500 volunteers, showed that anxiety and depression were significantly associated with the presence of IBS identified using the Manning criteria [26].

In a retrospective study [20] of patients selected by the modified criteria of Snape et al. [40] with a mean history of 3 years of IBS, the following psychosocial factors were associated with the presence of the disease: low income in large families; history of emotional or sexual abuse; home abandonment and infidelity; alcoholism; chronic diseases or disability; socioeconomic factors; unemployment, and drug addiction [20].

Diagnostic Criteria

So far there is no universally accepted biological marker for IBS and thus the disorder is positively diagnosed on the basis of a series of symptom criteria and limited diagnostic evaluation to exclude organic disease [41]. A consensus conference on IBS that took place in Rome in 1988, resulted in the development of diagnostic criteria (Rome '88) [42] and subsequently changes were made resulting in the Rome I criteria that were published in a book in 1994 [43]. The Rome I criteria have recently been reviewed and are now known as the Rome II criteria [44]. Of three discomfort/pain-related criteria (relieved by defecation, associated with a change in frequency of stools, associated with a change in form of stool), Rome II requires that patients have two instead of one, as does Rome I. Also, Rome II drops the Rome I requirement that patients must have two or more symptoms of altered bowel habits, bloating or mucus [44]. Furthermore, the Rome II committee suggests that subjects with functional bowel disorders may be divided into patients (those who had sought medical care for the functional bowel disorder) and non-patients (those who had never sought health care) [44]. These criteria have not yet been validated in Spanish.

In a preliminary study we analyzed the concordance of the Rome I and Rome II criteria in Mexican IBS patients [30]. Patients included were those previously diagnosed using the Rome I criteria in a tertiary referral academic center, and non-patients were those identified among healthy volunteers using a questionnaire that included both Rome I and Rome II criteria [30]. Although patients were significantly older compared to volunteers (43 vs. 29 years), there was a 71% concordance in patients and 75% concordance in non-patients between the Rome I and Rome II criteria [30]. It was concluded that the Rome I and Rome II criteria, translated into Spanish in Mexico, were highly concordant. We also confirmed that Rome II criteria in Spanish (Mexico) are more strict than the Rome I criteria as 100% of Rome II IBS patients and 88% of Rome II IBS non-patients were positive for the minimum of two bowel habit criteria required by the Rome I; conversely, only 75% of the Rome I IBS patients and 72% of Rome I IBS non-patients were positive for the minimum of the two pain-related criteria required by Rome II [30].

Symptom Subgroups Based on Predominant Bowel Habit

In a UCLA study, bowel habit predominance was 35% diarrhea, 22% constipation, and 43% alternating [45]. In a study from Olmstead County, Minnesota, it was 27% diarrhea, 27% constipation, 26% alternating and 20% could not be classified [46]. In our study, among Mexican IBS patients using the Rome I criteria, we found that 28% were diarrhea predominant, 25% constipation and 47% alternating [24], which was very similar to that reported in the USA studies [45, 46].

Physiological Studies

Physiological studies indicate the presence of visceral hypersensitivity as the most consistent abnormality in IBS [47–51]. Furthermore, IBS patients frequently relate their symptoms to food ingestion and a sensitization effect by food has been proposed [52].

In a physiological study among Mexican female patients with constipation predominant IBS, in which rectal balloon distension delivered by a barostat was used, it was shown that initial perception, gas and painful sensation thresholds were significantly decreased after food ingestion [28].

Capsaicin, the pungent ingredient of chili peppers, has been well characterized as a selective stimulant of unmyelinated C-fiber sensory afferent neurons, such as the peripheral terminals of spinal and vagal afferents [53]. Approximately 80% of C-fiber afferent neurons are polymodal 'silent' nociceptors that develop mechanosensitivity in relation to changes in the signal transduction mechanism of peripheral nerve terminals [53]. In Mexico, chili peppers are commonly part of the daily meal consumption. Recently we have finished a study among Rome I IBS patients that evaluated the rectal sensitivity thresholds to mechanical distension in response to a 1-week diet with or without guajillo chili peppers, using a randomized crossover study design [33]. During a tracking non-biased rectal distension protocol, we have found that 80% of our IBS patients were hypersensitive to discomfort threshold [33] using a cutoff point of 30 mm Hg as reported elsewhere [51]. No change was observed after 1 week of guajillo peppers in the diet. Conversely, a significant decrease in the rectal pain threshold during an ascending series of phasic distensions was observed [33].

It has been reported that a subgroup of constipation-predominant IBS patients have obstructive defecation [54]. In 1997 a Mexican study showed that patients with IBS were unable to widen the anorectal angle evaluated by defecography, claiming that IBS patients as a whole have pelvic-floor dysfunction [18]. This study included only what the authors considered to be 2 constipation-predominant patients and 13 patients who had normal frequency of defecation. The above suggests that the bowel habit predominance in this study was classified according to the frequency of bowel movements, and it is plausible to conclude that all patients included were constipation predominant with obstructive defecation based on the defecography findings. The same group of researchers found no correlation between transrectal ultrasonography, anorectal monometry and electromyography in 25 IBS patients with a mean age of 32 years [19].

Clinical Trials

In a recently published systematic review of randomized controlled trials of pharmacological treatments in IBS, smooth-muscle relaxants demonstrated clinical efficacy that was significantly better than placebo in patients with abdominal pain as the predominant symptom [55]. One of the studies included was conducted in Mexico and included 40 IBS patients who were allocated to 50 mg t.i.d. of pinaverium bromide versus placebo using a randomized study design [21]. Although the type of IBS according to predominant symptom was not reported, pinaverium bromide induced a significant improvement in abdominal pain, diminishing pain duration from several hours to minutes after food ingestion. Moreover, pinaverium bromide improved stool frequency and consistency, as well as anorectal symptoms [21]. The same group of researchers later demonstrated that pinaverium bromide induced an increase in the volume required to elicit the recto-anal inhibitory reflex [23]. The latter suggests an effect over colonic motility or an increase in rectal compliance [23].

Recently, α_2-agonist drugs have gained importance in the treatment of IBS [56]. Lidamidine hydrochloride, a peripheral α_2-receptor agonist used as an antidiarrheal medication has been tested in 40 Mexican Manning IBS patients [16]. In a controlled crossover design, patients were allocated to lidamidine vs. placebo and lidamidine plus psychotherapy vs. placebo plus psychotherapy. A superior global response was observed for lidamidine compared to placebo independent of the presence or absence of coadjuvant psychotherapy (94.7 vs. 68.4%, $p = 0.02$, and 84.3 vs. 63.2%, $p = 0.04$) [16]. No significant differences were found for individual symptoms such as abdominal pain or bloating [16]. In another study by the same group, both lidamidine and placebo significantly reduced symptom severity scores for pain severity and duration, distension and stool consistency, as well as increased sigmoid painful sensation to hand-held syringe distension [18]. The results of the latter study are controversial compared to the results in the previous one. Furthermore, according to the second study, both placebo and lidamidine seem to increase sigmoid sensitivity although it should be stated that painful sensation was evaluated with a syringe and not with a barostat which is the actual accepted method to evaluate visceral sensitivity.

Quality of Life Assessment

While monitoring patients, health-related quality of life (HRQOL) has become an important element in research and medical care [57]. The impact of IBS on the lifestyle of patients can be significant due to psychological distress and problems with sleep, work, leisure, diet, and sexual functioning, which results in increased health care use [58]. Thus, measurement of HRQOL is an important addition to the currently used outcome measurements in IBS. In a recent study using the SF-36 Health Survey, it has been shown that IBS patients had significantly worse HRQOL as compared to gastroesophageal reflux disease and diabetes mellitus. IBS patients had significantly better mental health scores than patients with depression, and worse bodily pain-related scores than dialysis-dependent end-stage renal disease patients [59].

By using the SF-36 Health Survey in Spanish and validated in Mexico [60], we have found [29] that IBS patients had significantly worse mental and physical summary scores as compared to patients with chronic hepatitis C and chronic pancreatitis. There was not any difference in any domain when IBS was compared to functional dyspepsia [29]. Of importance was the finding that IBS patients had a significantly higher score in bodily pain as compared to patients with chronic hepatitis C and chronic pancreatitis, which probably reflects the frequency and extent of role interference that is attributable to pain. Although the study included a small number of patients, the results hold strong after a strict Bonferroni correction [29].

Conclusions

In the current article we have reviewed 18 studies on IBS that were conducted in Mexico. Although most of the studies were published in abstract form, we can conclude that IBS in Mexico is similar to that reported in the international literature in terms of prevalence and gender distribution, impact of IBS on health care utilization, psychosocial factors, diagnostic criteria, bowel habit distribution and physiological findings.

Furthermore, some clinical and physiological trials are currently ongoing in Mexico. Little has been studied regarding extraintestinal symptoms and comorbidities associated with IBS such as fibromyalgia and more studies addressing this area are needed.

References

1 Drossman DA, Whitehead WE, Camilleri M: Irritable bowel syndrome: A technical review for practice guideline development. Gastroenterology 1997;112:2120–2137.
2 Camilleri M: Management of the irritable bowel syndrome. Gastroenterology 2001;120:652–668.
3 Mayer EA, Chang L, Lembo T: Brain-gut interactions: Implications for newer therapy. Eur J Surg 1998;582:50–55.
4 Schmulson M: Brain-gut interaction in irritable bowel syndrome: New findings of a multicomponent disease model. Isr Med Assoc J 2001;3:104–110.
5 Jinich H: Nuevas orientaciones en trastornos funcionales del aparato digestivo. Rev Gastroenterol Mex 1971;36:51–57.
6 Guevara L: Trastornos funcionales gastroduodenales. Rev Invest Clín 1971;23:221–235.
7 Snape WJ: Current concepts in the management of the irritable bowel syndrome. Rev Gastroenterol Mex 1994;59:127–132.
8 Jinich H: Enfermedad digestiva y padecer digestivo. Rev Gastroenterol Mex 1994;59:284–286.
9 Valdovinos Díaz MA: Síndrome de Intestino Irritable: ¿Trastorno Inflamatorio, Motor, Sensitivo o Psicológico? Rev Gastroenterol Mex 1996;61(suppl 2):43–44.
10 Villalobos PJ, Kershenobich D, Esquivel RF, Laviada AE, Laviada AA: Tratornos funcionales digestivos, estudio doble ciego con doxepin. Rev Gastroenterol Mex 1970;35:267–281.
11 Martín J, Awad RA, Camacho S, Santiago R: Correlación fisio-radiologica rectoanal en pacientes con síndrome de intestino Irritable. Rev Gastroenterol Mex 1992;57:260.
12 Nogueira JR, Mosqueda A: Consumo excesivo de alcohol en la población rural: aplicacion del cuestionario AUDIT y su correlación con factores socioeconómicos y síntomas de intestino irritable. Rev Gastroenterol Mex 1992;57:313.
13 Peniche A, Awad RA, Martínez P, Hernández A, Rivera JL, Ortiz F, Botey M: Correlación del dolor y la distension abdominal con la motilidad rectoanal en el síndrome de intestino irritable. Rev Gastroenterol Mex 1989;54:286.
14 Awad RA, Camacho S: Food influence rectal sensitivity in constipation predominant irritable bowel syndrome Latin patients. Gastroenterology 1999;116:A4151.
15 Awad R, Peniche A, Sanchez H, Botey M: Estudio aleatorio doble ciego controlado con placebo con aceite de menta piperita, respuesta electromecánica rectoanal a la comida en el síndrome de intestino irritable. Rev Gastroenterol Mex 1990;55:307.
16 Rodríguez A, Valdéz T, Llorens F: Tratamiento de colon irritable con lidamidina y psicoterapia de apoyo. Rev Gastroenterol Mex 1997;62:7–13.
17 Awad RA, Martin J, Cal y Major M, Noguera JL, et al: Transrectal ultrasonography: Relationship with anorectal manometry, electromyography and sensitivity tests in irritable bowel syndrome. Int J Colorectal Dis 1998;13:82–87.
18 Awad RA, Llorens F, Camelo AL, Sanchez M: A randomised double-blind placebo-controlled trial of lidamidine HCl in irritable bowel syndrome. Acta Gastroenterol Latinoam 2000;30:169–175.
19 Awad R, Martin J, Cal y Mayor M, Noguera JL, Ramos R, Amezcua C, Santiago R, Camacho S, Guevara M, Ramirez JL: Do anorectal parameters of ultrasonography, defecography, manometry, and electromyography correlate in irritable bowel syndrome? Gastroenterology 1996;110(suppl 1):A626.
20 Labastida H: Colon irritable. Rev Gastroenterol Mex 1982;47:24–29.
21 Awad RA, Dibildox M, Ortiz F: Irritable bowel syndrome treatment using pinaverium bromide as a calcium channel blocker. A randomized double-blind placebo-controlled trial. Acta Gastroenterol Latinoam 1995;25:137–144.
22 Awad RA, Martín J, Guevara M, Ramos R, Noguera JL, Camacho S, Santiago R: Defaecography in patients with irritable bowel syndrome and healthy volunteers. Int J Colorectal Dis 1997;12:91–94.
23 Awad RA, Cordova VH, Dibildox M, Santiago S: Reduction of post-prandial motility by pinaverium bromide a calcium channel blocker acting selectively on the gastrointestinal tract in patients with irritable bowel syndrome. Acta Gastroenterol Latinoam 1997;27:247–251.
24 Schmulson M, Valdovinos Díaz MA: Utilización de recursos médicos por los pacientes con síndrome de intestino irritable en un hospital de tercer nivel. Rev Gastroenterolol Mex 1998;63:6–10.
25 Modiano M, Harfush A, Hervella LM, Ciklik E, Villalobos JJ, Kershenobich D: Aspectos epidemiológicos de los trastornos funcionales digestivos. Rev Gastroenterol Mex 1982;47:302.
26 Mosqueta A, Nogueira JR: Epidemiología de los trastornos disfuncionales del tubo digestivo (intestino irritable) resultado de una encuesta aplicada en población rural abierta. Rev Gastroenterol Mex 1992;57(suppl 3):318.
27 Tanimoto MA, Schmulson M, Ramírez D: Prevalencia de los trastornos funcionales digestivos en estudiantes de medicina. Rev Gastroenterol Mex 1995;60(suppl 3):57.
28 Awad RA, Camacho S, Isidro L, Galvez E: A physiological response of rectal hypersensitivity is triggered after meals in female constipation predominant irritable bowel syndrome patients. Gastroenterology 2000;117(suppl 2):A5344.
29 Schmulson M, Robles G, Kershenobich D, López-Ridaura R, Hinojosa CA, Duarte CA, Bandera J: Los pacientes con trastornos funcionales digestivos (TFD) tienen mayor compromiso de la calidad de vida (CV) evaluada por el SF-36 comparados con pacientes con Hepatitis C y pancreatitis cónica. Rev Gastroenterol Mex 2000;65(Resúmenes):A50.
30 Morales G, Ocampo A, Valdovinos MA, Schmulson M: Concordancia entre los criterios de Roma I y Roma II para el diagnóstico del síndrome de colon irritable (SCI). Rev Gastroenterol Mex 2000;65(Resúmenes):A51.
31 Vázquez AI, Romero MR, Aguilar RJ: Trastornos del afecto. ¿Factor de riesgo para padecer trastornos funcionales digestivos? Rev Gastroenterol Mex 2000;65(Resúmenes):A51.
32 Bojórquez MC, Larrosa A, Martínez EO: Dolor abdominal crónico (DAC) en niños: ¿Síndrome de intestino irritable (SII) vs. dispepsia no ulcerosa (DNU)? Rev Gastroenterol Mex 2000;65(Resúmenes):A52.
33 Ocampo A, Schmulson M: El chile en la dieta disminuye el umbral sensorial rectal evaluado por barostato en pacientes con síndrome de colon irritable (SCI). Rev Gastroenterol Mex 2000;65(Resúmenes):A67.
34 Asociación Mexicana de Gastroenterología: Simposio: Trastornos funcionales del tubo digestivo (Resultado de la Encuesta Nacional). Rev Gastroenterol Mex 2000;65(Resúmenes):24–25.
35 Thompson WG, Creed FH, Drossman DA, Heaton K, Mazzacca G: Functional bowel disorders and functional abdominal pain; in Drossman D, Richter JE, Talley NJ, Thompson WG, Corazziari E, Whitehead WE (eds): The Functional Gastrointestinal Disorders, ed 1. Boston, Little Brown, 1994, pp 115–173.
36 Drossman DA, Li Z, Andruzzi E, et al: US householder survey of functional gastrointestinal disorders: Prevalence, sociodemography and health impact. Dig Dis Sci 1993;38:1569–1580.
37 Longstreth GF, Wolde-Isadik G: Irritable bowel-type symptoms in HMO examinees. Prevalence, demographics and clinical correlates. Dig Dis Sci 1993;9:1581–1589.
38 Drossman DA, McKee DC, Sandler RS, Mitchell CM, Cramer EM, Lowman BC, Burger AL: Psychosocial factors in the irritable bowel syndrome. Gastroenterology 1988;95:701–708.
39 Whitehead WE, Bosmajian L, Zonderman A, Costa PT, Schuster MM: Role of psychological symptoms in irritable bowel syndrome: Comparison of community and clinical samples. Gastroenterology 1988;95:709–714.
40 Snape WJ Jr, Carlson GM, Matarrazo SA, Cohen S: Evidence that abnormal myoelectrical activity produces colonic motor dysfunction in the bowel syndrome. Gastroenterology 1977;72:383–387.

41 Schmulson M, Chang L: Diagnostic approach to the patients with irritable bowel syndrome. Am J Med 1999;107:20S–26S.
42 Thompson WG, Dotevall G, Drossman DA, Heaton KW, Kruis W: Irritable bowel syndrome: Guidelines for the diagnosis. Gastroenterol Int 1989;2:92–95.
43 Thompson WG, and the Working Team for Functional Bowel Disorders: Functional bowel disorders and functional abdominal pain; in Drossman DA, Richter JE, Talley NJ, Thompson WG, Corazziari E, Whitehead WE (eds): The Functional Gastrointestinal Disorders, ed 1. Boston, Little Brown, 1994.
44 Thompson WG, Longstreth GF, Drossman DA, Heaton KW, Irvine EJ, Müller-Lissner SA: Functional bowel disorders and functional abdominal pain. Gut 1999;45(suppl 2):II43–II47.
45 Schmulson M, Lee OY, Chang L, Naliboff B, Mayer EA: Symptom differences in moderate to severe IBS patients on predominant bowel habit. Am J Gastroenterol 1999;94:2929–2935.
46 Talley NJ, Zinsmeister AR, Melton J: Irritable bowel syndrome in a community: Symptom subgroups, risk factors, and health care utilization. Am J Epidemiol 1995;142:76–83.
47 Ritchie J: Pain from distension of the pelvic colon by inflating a balloon in the irritable bowel syndrome. Gut 1973;14:125–132.
48 Prior A, Maxton DG, Whorwell PJ: Anorectal manometry in irritable syndrome: Differences between diarrhoea and constipation predominant subjects. Gut 1990;31:458–462.
49 Mertz H, Naliboff B, Munakata J, Niazi N, Mayer EA: Altered rectal perception is a biological marker of patients with irritable bowel syndrome. Gastroenterology 1995;109:40–52.
50 Lembo T, Mukanata J, Naliboff B, Fullerton S, Mayer EA: Sigmoid afferent mechanisms in patients with irritable bowel syndrome. Dig Dis Sci 1997;42:1112–1120.
51 Schmulson M, Chang L, Naliboff B, Lee OY, Mayer EA: Correlation of symptom criteria with perception thresholds during rectosigmoid distension in irritable bowel syndrome patients. Am J Gastroenterol 2000;95:152–156.
52 Dainese R, Galliani EA, De Lazzari F, Di Leo V, Naccarato R: Discrepancies between reported food intolerance and sensitization test findings in irritable bowel syndrome patients. Am J Gastroenterol 1999;94:1892–1897.
53 Mayer EA, Gebhart GF: Functional bowel disorders and the visceral hyperalgesia hypothesis; in Mayer EA, Raybould HE (eds): Basic and Clinical Aspects of Chronic Abdominal Pain, ed 1. Amsterdam, Elsevier, 1993, vol 9, pp 3–28.
54 Mertz H, Naliboff B, Mayer EA: Physiology of refractory chronic constipation. Am J Gastroenterol 1999;94:609–615.
55 Jailwala J, Imperiale TF, Kroenke K: Pharmacologic treatment of the irritable bowel syndrome: A systematic review of randomized, controlled trials. Ann Intern Med 2000;133: 136–147.
56 Bharucha AE, Camilleri M, Zinsmeister AR, Hanson RB: Adrenergic modulation of human colonic motor and sensory function. Am J Physiol 1997;273:G997–G1006.
57 Yacavone RF, Locke GR-III, Provenzale DT, Eisen GM: Quality of life measurement in gastroenterology: What is available. Am J Gastroenterol 2001;96:285–297.
58 Farmer RG, Easley KA, Farmer JM: Quality of life assessment by patients with inflammatory bowel disease. Cleve Clin J Med 1992;59:35–42.
59 Gralnek IM, Hays RD, Kilbourne A, Naliboff B, Mayer EA: The impact of irritable bowel syndrome on health related quality of life. Gastroenterology 2000;19:654–660.
60 Zuniga MA, Carrillo-Jimenez GT, Fos PJ, Gandek B, Medina-Moreno MR: Evaluación del estado de salud con la Encuesta SF-36: resultados preliminares en México. Salud Pública Méx 1999;41:110–118.

Digestive Diseases

Author Index

Subject Index

KARGER
Fax + 41 61 306 12 34
E-Mail karger@karger.ch
www.karger.com

Accessible online at:
www.karger.com/journals/ddi